REDOX CELL
SIGNALING

Redox Cell Signaling

HOW YOUR BODY TALKS

Stan M. Gardner, MD, CNS

Pocket Garden Press

Contents

Copyright

Prologue

Dear Reader:

In writing this book, I wanted to make the rather complicated concepts of Redox signaling simple and easy to understand. Most of us are not scientists. Most of us have experienced incredible health benefits from using Redox products, and want to be able to explain the amazing benefits of Redox signaling so that others can understand them. I've included lots of pictures in the text to make concepts visual and understandable.   As you read this, it may be helpful for you to know that:

1. I'm a medical doctor of over 45 years.

2. I'm a Certified Nutrition Specialist, also board certified in Anti-Aging and Regenerative Medicine.

3. I'm not a writer by training, so you'll have to deal with that.

With all of that out of the way, let's get started:

Every few decades in the health arena, a discovery occurs that revolutionizes the health field landscape. A few examples:

Vitamin C

Sailors on long voyages were prone to getting scurvy, an illness caused by vitamin C deficiency, from the 15th to 18th centuries. An estimated two million seamen died of scurvy's lethal effects during those years—three times as many as the number of soldiers who died in the American Civil War.

Scientists discovered signs of scurvy in the bones of La Isabella settlement (now Dominican Republic) founded by Christopher Columbus in 1494. The book *Moby Dick* also describes symptoms of scurvy.

While today, most of us are famiiar with the health benefits of vitamins, such knowledge was not common among the common people--or even the "experts." Vitamin C is necessary to produce collagen, the connective tissue that keeps the body together. Without collagen, the body disintegrates, the skin breaks down into blisters and ulcers, the gums putrefy and turn black, and previously broken bones re-break and old wounds open up. The nervous system also breaks down, because vitamin C scavenges free radicals (oxidants). Without this support, oxidation occurs. Oxidation destroys neurotransmitter effectiveness. If vitamin C is missing, the brain starts hallucinating.

James Lind was a naval physician who saw the ravages of scurvy first hand for years. In 1747 he performed the first recorded medical trial--ever. He took 12 sailors with advanced scurvy aboard a ship. He divided them into six groups of two. With each group he administered one of six recommended treatments for scurvy. The only pair that improved substantially were given two oranges and one lemon each day.

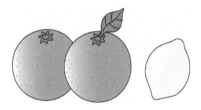

It took an additional 46 years before the Admiralty of England issued an order providing lemon juice to all sailors, making it possible for this horrible disease to finally be cured.

Unfortunately, long implementation delays tend to be a pattern with most medical breakthroughs.

Albert Szent-Györgyi came from a long line of scientists who went into research after receiving medical degrees. After years of painstaking effort and study, he was able to isolate vitamin C from paprika in 1933, for which he received the Nobel Prize 4 years later. Scurvy is seen only rarely now.[1]

Vitamin B1 (Thiamine)

In the 1800s, Europeans colonized Asia and brought with them steam-powered machines that completely polished rice. Polished rice was supposed to be superior to unpolished rice, and certainly was preferred by the rich who could afford it. Within a few years, beriberi was rampant in Japan.

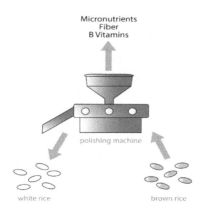

Beriberi manifests as either a heart and circulatory system failure or nerve damage, leading to loss of muscle strength, and even paralysis.

Kanehiro Takaki, surgeon general of the Japanese Imperial Navy, noticed a connection between the sailors' diets and the development of beriberi. By substituting white rice with barley, vegetables, fish and meat, the navy eliminated beriberi within 6 years.

At this same time, the Dutch Indies was having a crippling endemic of beriberi. Christiaan Eijkman, a Dutch microbiologist, had the theory that beriberi was an infectious disease. He tried to infect chickens with material from two chickens that died of beriberi. It did not work, but he did notice that even chickens that had no contact with beriberi chickens got the disease.

The cook had been feeding the chickens leftover polished rice from the hospital. When the replacement cook refused to feed the chickens leftover polished rice, but fed them raw unpolished rice, beriberi disappeared. He concluded that the unpolished rice contained an antidote to the bacterial toxin, the anti-beriberi factor.

It wasn't until 1906 that Frederick Hopkins demonstrated there were accessory factors in food that were necessary to maintain good health. In 1912 a Polish biochemist, Casimir Funk, thought he had isolated the anti-beriberi factor, which he named a *vital amine*, or vitamin. In 1926 researchers isolated the anti-beriberi factor from rice bran extracts. Thiamine, or vitamin B1, is the "factor" that prevents beriberi. In 1929, Hopkins and Eijkman were awarded the Nobel Prize in Physiology for the discovery of vitamins.

Even with this revolutionary breakthrough, modern medicine still struggles with how to apply this valuable information in the clinical setting.[2, 3]

Penicillin

Alexander Fleming was a Professor of Bacteriology at St. Mary's Hospital in London in the 1920s. He had a set of petri dishes containing colonies of Staphylococcus. This organism killed 80% of people who got infected with it. And there was no treatment for it.

Upon returning home from a vacation in 1928 he noticed something different in one of the petri dishes. A mold was growing in one, and the Staphylococcus organism could not survive near it. He discovered this "mold juice" also killed other organisms, including streptococcus, meningococcus and diphtheria bacillus.

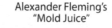

Alexander Fleming's
"Mold Juice"

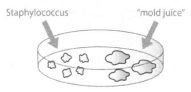

Eleven years later, Howard Florey and Ernst Chain and colleagues from the School of Pathology at Oxford University were able to stabilize it. They began animal experiments and tried to make enough for further experimentation.

Albert Alexander, a 43-year old policeman, was the first human to receive penicillin. He scratched his face while pruning roses, and soon developed life-threatening boils and abscesses on his face and lungs. After only a few days on the drug he had a miraculous recovery, but the medicine ran out before completing a course of it, and he subsequently died.

The production of penicillin remained inadequate to treat most of the people that needed it. During World War II treating afflicted soldiers was the highest priority. In 1945, adequate production was sufficient to make it available to the general public. Millions of lives have been saved with the use of penicillin as an antibiotic against susceptible bacterial organisms.[4]

Antioxidants

Antioxidants were used in the rubber industry in the late 19th century to slow down degeneration of rubber. In the 1920s, antioxidants were used in the food industry to slow down the degradation of food, but no one had figured out the exact mechanism (oxidation/reduction) by which the slowdown occurred.

In the 1950s, two Buenos Aires researchers, Rebecca and Daniel Gilbert found that radiation produced much greater damage when in the presence of oxygen. Thus began the identification of *free radicals* and the start of chain reactions involving oxygen.[5]

Redox Technology

In the early 2000s a biotech company invested tens of millions of dollars researching a product involving signaling molecules, without exactly knowing what the active ingredient was. When the company's funding ran out, the principals of the company asked businessman Verdis Norton to join the board of this company so they could hopefully find funds to keep the research going. But it was too late: with $1M in debt and on the verge of bankruptcy, they decided to sell off the assets of the company, including the signaling molecules technology.

Verdis decided to buy the part he was most interested in—the signaling molecules technology, noting that it achieved great health benefits. One year later the mechanism of action of these molecules was identified as *redox biochemistry*. At that time the molecule could only be made in a small desktop machine and the active Redox molecules lasted just a few minutes before they degraded.

Verdis gathered a team of researchers and tasked them with stabilizing the product to extend the efficacy and life of the molecules. The researchers were able to create stabilized redox signaling molecules. When the product was given to 40 people with various health conditions, some remarkable results were noted, including a few whose lives dramatically improved as a result of this discovery.

Verdis discussed various distribution models with colleagues. A pharmaceutical company looked at the research and wanted to buy the formula with the stipulation that Verdis and others would no longer use it to help people with their health. This condition raised concerns:

> What will happen to the people on the product whose lives are enhanced if we can no longer provide it?

> It would take years of going through FDA regulation protocols before the pharmaceutical company could get it to market.

The chance also existed that because of the widespread benefits of the technology, the pharmaceutical company would buy the revolutionary health patents and bury them. The technology would then never hit the market.

With those concerns, Verdis Norton refused to sell to the pharmaceutical company and instead decided to create his own company to distribute the product through direct sales. The name of the company became ASEA, which did a soft launch in July 2009, and more formally in September 2010. They are the only company in the world with this Redox technology and the patents to protect it.[6]

This book is about the revolutionary potential that REDOX molecules bring to our health and life.

Chapter Notes

1. Sion Worrall, A Nightmare Disease Haunted Ships During Age of Discovery. (National Geographic, 2017), 01.
2. Michelle Schneider and Norman Egger, MD, History of a Vitamin (The Hospitalist, 2006 November), 11.
3. Chitra Badii and Matthew Solan and Lauren Reed-Guy, Beriberi (Medically reviewed by Debra Rose Wilson, PhD MSN RN on April 12, 2017) https://www.health-line.com/health/beriberi//causes.
4. Discovery and Development of Penicillin (American Chemical Society International Historic Chemical Landmarks) http://www.acs.org/content/acs/en/education/whatischemistry/landmarks/flemingpenicillin.html (accessed 2020).
5. History of Antioxidants, https://www.antiaging-club.it/en/News/HISTORY-OF-ANTIOXI-DANTS.html?RwPag=true&pagina_ID=565.
6. Author's personal observation from presentations and interviews since 2011.

1

REDOX Defined

REDOX refers to a change of state in a molecule. This change in state causes a change in the shape (structure), the function or activity of that molecule. It may turn it "on" or "off." It may change the rate of a reaction, or may even make the reaction happen. This change in state repairs cells. It also can cause the death of cells that are beyond repair.

All this and more is what REDOX is about. You can use your knowledge about REDOX to enhance your health and your life.

What is REDOX? Where did the term come from? What does it mean?

REDOX combines parts of two words—RED from REDuction and OX from OXidation.

We'll go over the OXidation part of this combination first by observing the chemical reaction of oxygen to iron in the air. If metal iron is not protected by paint, a chemical reaction of iron metal with oxygen in the air causes iron to "oxidize" or rust.

The same thing happens when the protective covering of a banana is peeled back, or an apple is cut and no longer has a peel to protect the fruit inside. The oxygen in the air chemically combines with the fruit and "oxidizes" it. The fruit turns brown, meaning it has "oxidized" or is in an "oxidized" state.

Oxidation

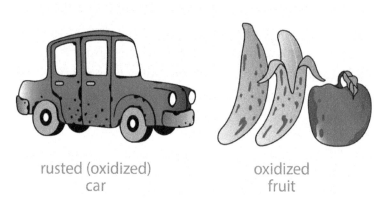

rusted (oxidized)
car

oxidized
fruit

Similar REDOX reactions take place millions of times each second in our 75 trillion cells. However, in our body oxygen is not the only factor in these reactions. Electrons and hydrogen also exchange between molecules. Each of these exchanges changes the state of the molecules, also called the "oxidative state" of the molecule.

When a molecule donates its oxygen molecule to another

molecule, the process is oxidation. The molecule with the extra oxygen is in the oxidized state, just as "iron rust" means the iron is oxidized, or in the oxidized state. When the oxidized molecule gives up the extra oxygen, it is no longer oxidized, but is in a reduced state. The reduced state of the molecule tends to be more stable. More stable means the molecule is no longer causing damage to other cells.

Molecules that have 1) oxygen as the donor and 2) are capable of donating it are called *reactive oxygen species (ROS)*. Those types of molecules that have oxygen, but do not donate it, are not ROS. Although this book focuses on ROS, there are molecules with nitrogen and sulfur that are also reactive, called *reactive nitrogen species (RNS)* and *reactive sulfur species (RSS)*. Like ROS, they can both act as signaling molecules and can affect tissue, which I'll explain.

Transfer of electrons between molecules is different from transfer of oxygen. When a stable molecule gives up an electron, its state changes to an oxidized state, which is un-stable. However, this instability is what gives it the ability to signal other cells and make things happen. Basically, its instability sends out the message that it needs a donation. When another molecule donates its electron back to the oxidized molecule, the oxidized molecule is reduced and becomes stable. Of course, the molecule which donated its electron has now oxidized.

We can liken this exchange to a person who has money. The wealthy person wants to transfer it to someone who does not have money. After the transfer, the person who had money no longer has money, and the person without money now has money. Maybe that's the reason for an unstable economy!

Redox

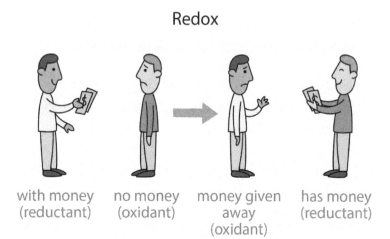

with money	no money	money given	has money
(reductant)	(oxidant)	away	(reductant)
		(oxidant)	

Some of the molecules produced in REDOX are better at cell signaling. Others are poor at cell signaling and do damage to the cells and body. An oxidized molecule causes damage in its search for an electron, pinging around rather frantically in the body. We might compare it to a hard metal ball thrown repeatedly against a soft wood surface, leaving dents and dings in the wood. An oxidized molecule wants to become stable again in the reduced state. You can imagine the reduced state as a happy state with a smiley face on it.

Redox

"Oxidant"
free radical
missing
electron

"Reductant"
reduced state
electron
full

The oxidized state is unstable and anxious, with an anxious face on it. We call the oxidized molecules *free radicals*. When free radicals exist in abundance, they cause the damage that we call *oxidative stress*.

Some of the oxidized free radicals last a fraction of a second before they are reduced. Other free radicals last for many seconds before they are reduced. They could actually move to a different area from where they were formed. Still other free radicals are less reactive and cause less damage.

In summary:

- REDOX refers to a change in state of a molecule from a reduced state (stable, "happy") to an oxidized state (unstable, "anxious"). This change back and forth happens over and over again.

- Some oxidized molecules function in signaling the cell to do certain things, and then the molecule is reduced to shut it off.

- Some oxidized molecules cause damage to the cells and tissues and need to be reduced before they cause too much damage.

Looking ahead:

Chapter Two talks about the specifics of cell signaling in various tissues of the body.

Chapter Three explores the sources of oxidized molecules both inside and outside the body.

Chapter Four focuses on the mechanism inside the body to squelch the oxidation process.

These critical mechanisms permit balance in the REDOX process.

Chapter Five addresses the damage in cells and in the body when ROS is excessive and out of balance, called *oxidative stress.*

Chapters Six, Seven, and Eight provide solutions we are all looking for to use these cells to our best advantage, to have a healthy REDOX life.

Chapters Two through Five are a synthesis and simplification of various parts of AS Naidu's book, REDOX Life published in August 2013. If the science in the next four chapters is too laborious to understand, jump ahead to

Chapter Six to learn how to use REDOX principles in your life to be a healthier you.

2

Cell Signaling from REDOX Reactions

Gene Regulation

The nucleus of each cell houses our chromosomes, 23 pair or 46 chromosomes in humans. A chromosome is made up of DNA, with a protein scaffolding for support. DNA stores information, which the cell uses to maintain structure in the cell or perform functions within the cell.

If the body needs to make an antioxidant protein, how does that take place? First of all, systems within the cell sense the ROS status. An elevation of certain ROS molecules (O_2^-, H_2O_2, lipid hydroperoxides, or other RNS molecules) activates a protein on the chromosome. This initiates the process of *gene transcription*. Transcribing a gene is like transcribing or copying notes from a class into a form that is readable and easy to understand. *Transcribing* a gene is making a copy of the gene so that a message can go to the "factory" in the body for production.

Transcription of DNA to make new product

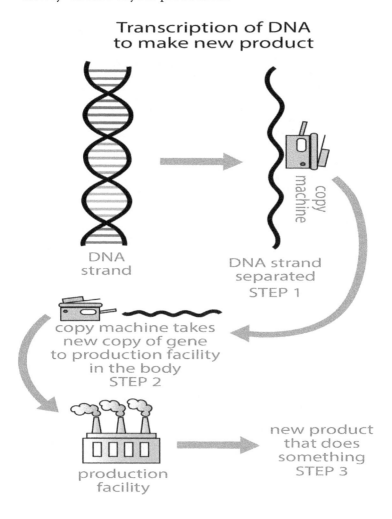

DNA strand

DNA strand separated
STEP 1

copy machine

copy machine takes new copy of gene to production facility in the body
STEP 2

production facility

new product that does something
STEP 3

The cell makes at least 80 different substances to protect itself from ROS damage.

Other genes stop the cell from dividing, so that repair can take place. Some genes that ROS triggers initiate cell death, called *programmed cell death* or *apoptosis*. Clean-up crews (*macrophages*) come in to remove and digest the dead cell parts for recycling.[1]

Protein/Enzyme Regulation

Proteins are made up of 20 (or 21 or 22, depending on who is counting) amino acids, of which nine are essential; that is, they have to be consumed into the body because the body cannot make them. One amino acid, cysteine, is very easy to oxidize because it has a sulfur group on it. Some other amino acids--such as methionine, tyrosine and tryptophan-- are much more difficult to oxidize.

Cysteine is like a molecular switch. *"Cystine"* is the oxidized form of cysteine. When cysteine is oxidized, the switch turns on and any number of actions may take place. In the nucleus, through the formation of hydrogen peroxide (H_2O_2) or RNS molecule *nitric oxide* (NO), the following may take place because of the oxidized cysteine:

- DNA repair

- Chromosome stability

- Gene transcription

- Cell division ceases

- Cell death triggered

An example of how an amino acid changes
through oxidation to perform different tasks.

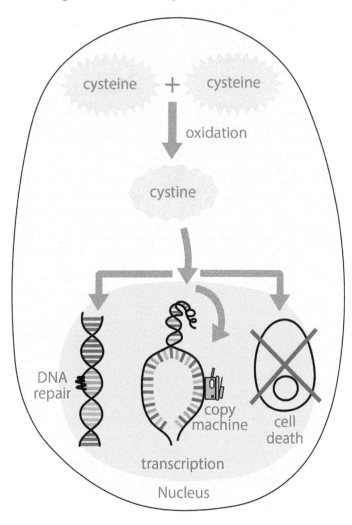

Outside the nucleus, the oxidized *cystine* may:

- form a bond between sulfur units (disulfide bond). Disulfide bonds stabilize the 3-dimensional shape of proteins, or form the connection between proteins. Electrons are released in this process. The released electrons are used to reduce oxidized molecules. Antibodies need these bonds in order to function. So do insulin chains. Without these bonds, the protein cannot function.

- further oxidize into *sulfinic* or *sulfonic acid*. Sulfinic acid is the reduced form of the oxidized sulfonic acid. One-electron transfers of sulfinic acid take place in the chemical process to produce *surfactants*. Surfactants are used in cleaning detergents to improve spreading and wetting ability.

- bind with nitrogen to make a sulfonamide. This is one of many categories of antibiotic, which includes the widely known Bactrim.

Any of these three reactions changes the structure (form) or function of the protein. This may affect metabolism, cell signaling or antioxidant defense pathways.

Enzymes are proteins that accelerate chemical reactions in cells. Enzyme activation may take place through oxidation, through cysteine, or through another process that places a phosphate molecule (PO_4^{3-}) on the enzyme. Which enzyme is activated determines the function or reaction that takes place. If the protease enzyme, *caspase*, is activated, pro-grammed cell death *(apoptosis)* could take place. Apoptosis is needed to replace damaged or worn out cells.

In addition to the amino acid cysteine, *methionine* has a sulfur molecule that can be oxidized or form a sulfide-to-sulfide double bond. *Proline* and *arginine* can be changed with the addition of an ^-OH group or *tyrosine* can have nitrogen added to it. All of these changes to these protein amino acids affect their shape, stability or function, and are mediated through REDOX processes. These changes in REDOX signaling affect the:

- ability of receptors on the cell wall to function

- transporter proteins, helping them to do their job

- enzymes, to move chemical reactions forward

- gene transcription initiation and building of new material in the cell

- structure of proteins that contract or cause movement.[2]

Mitochondria

The mitochondria is called the "powerhouse" of the cell,

because it produces energy (ATP-Adenosine triphosphate) for the cell. The number of mitochondria in the cell depends on the energy needs of that cell. Muscles, especially the heart muscle, have thousands of mitochondria in each cell. Red blood cells don't have any mitochondria.

The major pathway of ATP production is called the *electron transport chain.* This nine-step pathway, along with the enzymes that drive it, is found at the inner mitochondrial membrane. A massive movement of electrons takes place in this pathway. Most of the oxidation and reduction in this pathway ends up with water and oxygen as end products. However, 1% to 2% of the oxidized product escapes from the mitochondria in the form of ROS, reactive oxygen species.

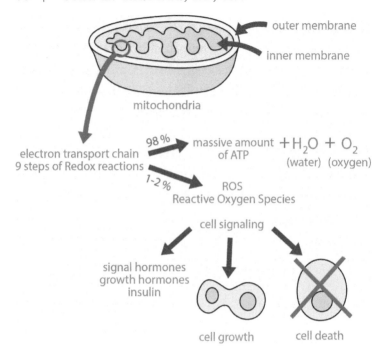

ROS molecules function as cell signaling molecules. The hormones of the body work, nutrients are utilized and oxygen use is regulated at normal levels of hydrogen peroxide. ROS signaling molecules also modulate cell growth and death, energy production and metabolism (the processes of the cell that keep it functioning). If the mitochondria are not functioning normally, or they have been damaged, the result is decreased ATP production and increased ROS molecules. This may contribute to oxidative stress in the body, rather than more cell signaling.[3]

Vascular Regulation

The vascular system is comprised of the arteries (which take blood from the heart to the body by means of the heart pumping), capillaries (where exchange of nutrients and waste products takes place) and veins (which return blood to the heart by skeletal muscle movement and one-way valves).

Arteries have a wall of connective tissue on the outside of the blood vessel wall to prevent it from rupturing. Inside that layer in an artery is a muscle layer which constricts (makes smaller) or relaxes (makes the blood vessel bigger). The inside layer of the artery is a single layer of cells called the *endothelium*. Signaling takes place in the endothelial lining. The signaling determines blood pressure and smooth transport of nutrients and waste products.

The transfer of oxygen and nutrients from the blood into the body takes place in the capillaries. There are holes in the capillaries, which permit the nutrients and oxygen from the arteries to go into the tissue. The waste products from the tissue get into the blood for delivery, through the veins, to the lungs and kidneys for removal from the body.

Although RNS with nitric oxide is a huge factor in blood vessel function, ROS also plays a role. The formation of new blood vessels, called *angiogenesis*, needs cell signaling from oxygen (O_2^-) and hydrogen peroxide (H_2O_2), to trigger growth factors. One of these growth factors is called *vascular endothelial growth factor* (VEGF) and is activated by ROS which initiates the process of blood vessel formation and tube formation.[4]

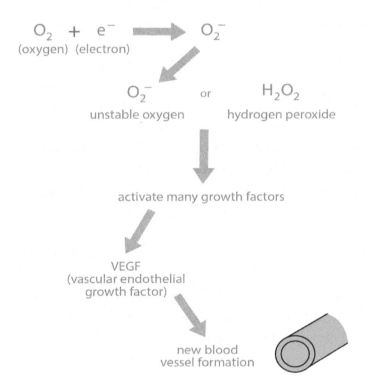

Two Reactive Oxygen Species (ROS) that Participate in Cell Signaling

O_2 + e^- ⟶ O_2^-
(oxygen) (electron)

O_2^- or H_2O_2
unstable oxygen   hydrogen peroxide

activate many growth factors

VEGF
(vascular endothelial
growth factor)

new blood
vessel formation

Immune Regulation

The immune system is composed of two parts. One part is an immediate inflammatory response to any foreign sub-

stance identified by the body. These inflammatory molecules attract white cells in an effort to identify the enemy
and kill it. This general response is called the *innate system.*
This system is activated whenever we cut or scrape our-
selves. Soon after the cut takes place, the immediate, non-
specific immune cells are attracted to the area and cause
redness (inflammation) and pain. The immune cells initiate
the repair process in the body.

The other part of the immune system is specific toward a
unique organism. The immune system responses can be
mounted against chicken pox virus or diphtheria bacteria.
They take about two weeks to form, are called antibodies,
and are formed upon initial exposure to the organism. An
army of these antibodies is just waiting for the same exposure to enter the body so it can fight it immediately and
quickly. This system is called the *acquired system.*

What is the trigger for these reactions to take place? It is the
ROS oxygen (O_2^-) and hydrogen peroxide (H_2O_2). They,
along with other signaling molecules, cause nuclear factor
kappa B (NF_KB) to activate the transcription of over 100
genes as part of these innate and acquired systems. These
genes are triggers of the inflammatory response and assist in
the killing of unwanted cells and microbes.[5]

Immune System activation through ROS

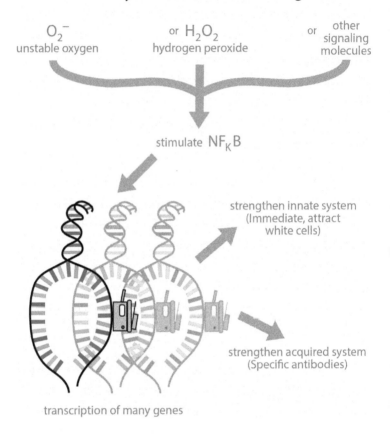

O_2^-
unstable oxygen

or H_2O_2
hydrogen peroxide

or other
signaling
molecules

stimulate NF_KB

strengthen innate system
(Immediate, attract
white cells)

strengthen acquired system
(Specific antibodies)

transcription of many genes

Phagocytes and Respiratory Burst

Oxygen is brought into the body with each inhalation (breathing in) while waste products like carbon dioxide are exhaled (breathing out). There is no storage form for oxygen in the body. Mitochondria forms ninety-eight percent of the inhaled oxygen into ATP *(adenosine tryphosphate)*.

Phagocytes is the broad term for several white blood cells (*neutrophils, lymphocytes, eosinophils, phagocytes*) that kill foreign microbes upon their entering the body. They do this by making toxic ROS molecules that serve as bullets to "kill" the microbes. When needed, phagocytes increase their oxygen consumption so they can make more oxidized ROS to "kill" the microbes. This rise in oxygen consumption is called *respiratory burst*, and is part of the innate (non-specific) immune system.

Oxygen consumption produces several ROS by-products of this oxygen consumption. Oxidized O_2^- and hydrogen peroxide (H_2O_2) are bullets that mainly kill foreign microbes, without injuring local cells.

How ROS Maintains the Health of the Body

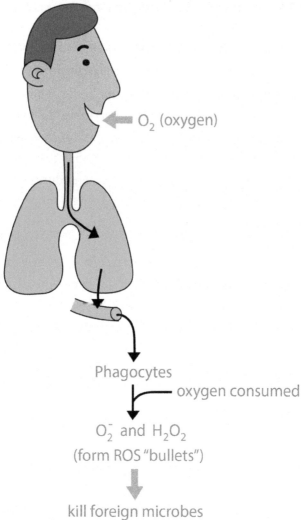

O_2 (oxygen)

Phagocytes

oxygen consumed

O_2^- and H_2O_2
(form ROS "bullets")

kill foreign microbes

There are other ROS that kill microbes. The addition of chlorite (Cl^-) produces hypochlorite (OCl^-), which is toxic to both microbes and normal cells. Certain metals assist in the conversion of H_2O_2 into ^-OH, which kills microbes but may also cause damage to DNA, protein, lipids, and sugars. These more toxic substances need to be quickly neutralized by antioxidants like melatonin, glutathione, and vitamin E.

Phagocytes naturally produce ozone (O_3). Ozone (O_3) is also a powerful anti-microbial while preserving the health of normal cells.[6]

Apoptosis

When a cell is damaged enough that it is beyond repair, the cell has several mechanisms to self-destruct. This eliminates non-functioning cells, so as to keep the cell-to-cell (inter-cellular) function intact in tissues and organs. It also does not permit damaged cells that may be harmful to the body to multiply. Apoptosis is the most efficient process for cell death, compared to other processes like necrosis. Apoptosis is the natural process for cell death that does not damage nearby cells. Necrosis causes local cell damage after the cell dies, and is triggered by trauma or infection.

Within the cell membrane are a myriad of receptors, transporters, channels and various ways of transmitting messages across the membrane to the inside of the cell. One of these is a death-inducing signaling complex, which activates *caspase* enzymes inside the cell. The initiator caspases start the death process, followed by activation of the executioner caspases. These executioner caspases are enzymes that breakdown cell membranes and destroy the contents of the cell so they don't damage surrounding cells when they die. Garbage truck crews (*macrophages*) come in and clean up the mess.

What is the trigger that initiates this death inducing signaling complex? Excessive oxidation outside the cell activates other proteins (TNF, FasL) and death receptors (DR4, DR5) to trigger the death-inducing signaling complex at the cell membrane.

Apoptosis (cell destruction) from Stressors Outside Cell

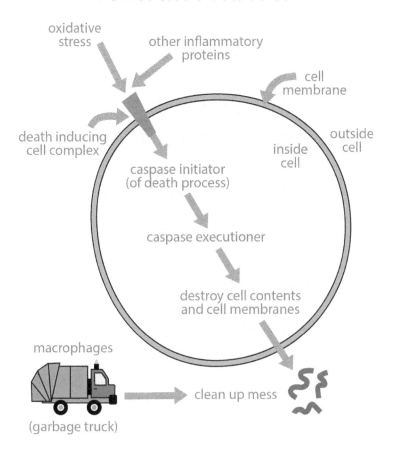

A separate mechanism to initiate apoptosis occurs inside the cell. When the oxidative levels rise too high inside the cell, the mitochondrial DNA gets damaged. The membrane around the mitochondria opens up and releases *cytochrome c*, one of the components of the electron transport chain. Cytochrome c combines with an apoptotic protease enzyme to trigger the initiator caspases as noted above. This separate mechanism causes apoptosis through the executioner caspases as above.[7]

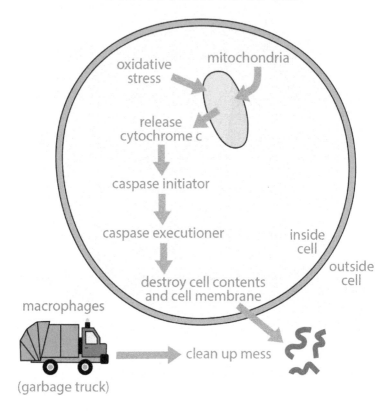

Apoptosis (cell destruction) from Stressors Inside Cell

oxidative stress

mitochondria

release cytochrome c

caspase initiator

caspase executioner

inside cell

outside cell

destroy cell contents and cell membrane

macrophages

clean up mess

(garbage truck)

Thus, REDOX shows itself once again to be a major mechanism to signal cells to perform their various functions —metabolism, energy production, repair and death of cells, differentiation of new cells, defenses and protection of cells.

Chapter Notes

1. A S Naidu, "REDOX Signaling: Gene Regulation," in *REDOX Life* (Pamona, California: Bio-Rep Network, 2013), 172-175.
2. Naidu, "Protein/Enzyme Regulation," 176-178.
3. Naidu, "Mitochondrial Regulation," 179-181.
4. Naidu, "Vascular Regulation," 182-185.
5. Naidu, "Immune Regulation," 186-187.
6. Naidu, "Phagocytes," 126-127.
7. Naidu, "Apoptosis," 188-190.

3

Sources of Oxidized Molecules (ROS)

How many ways does our body make and get exposed to ROS molecules? The number is almost endless. Here they are categorized into those exposures from outside the body and inside the body that form ROS.

Exposures from Outside the Body

Radiation and X-rays (medical X-rays and CAT scans, UV rays from the sun, scanners at airports) trigger the formation of ^-OH free radicals,[1] which is more damaging to other cells and has less signaling capability.

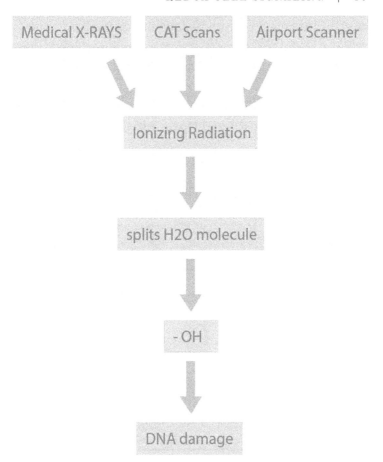

An endless number of chemical pollutants are introduced into the air and environment, with more being added almost daily. Pesticides and herbicides produce free radicals, and many people who use them do not use adequate protection. We face toxic exposures at the gasoline pump, with vehicle emissions, and waste from rendering plants. Asbestos produces ROS and can still be found in walls of old homes. We also find toxic substances in the water, including chlorine, fluoride, arsenic, lead, chemical fertilizer, bisphenol A.

Poisons (Toxins) Outside the Home that Create Free Radicals (ROS)

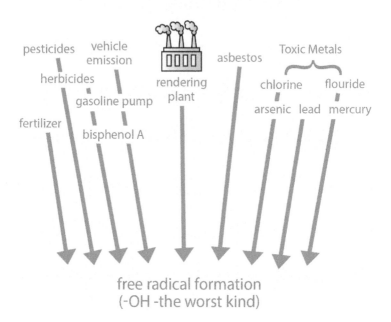

pesticides · vehicle emission · herbicides · gasoline pump · fertilizer · bisphenol A · rendering plant · asbestos · Toxic Metals · chlorine · flouride · arsenic · lead · mercury

free radical formation
(-OH -the worst kind)

Cigarette smoke is among the most toxic exposures frequently inhaled, with greater than 100,000,000,000,000 (10^{14}) ROS toxic elements with each inhalation.

Harmful Effects of Smoking

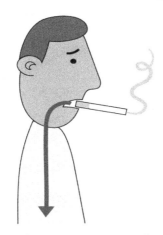

more than 100,000,000,000,000 free
radicals absorbed per inhalation

Petroleum-based products like paint and furniture polish contain toluene, benzene and formaldehyde, all of which contribute to the ROS load.

The air in our homes is another source of toxicity. Chemicals are released with the outgassing of new furniture, carpets, and new paint. Clothes brought in from dry cleaning release chemicals. Many personal care products are toxic—fingernail polish and remover, hair spray, aftershave, perfume. Even scented candles and air fresheners are laden with chemicals. As if these were not enough, shampoos, lotions, toothpaste and mouthwash all have chemicals that add to the toxic load. Because our homes tend to be sealed to reduce heat and air conditioning leaks, these chemicals are trapped in our houses.

Personal Care Products in Home that create Free Radicals (ROS)

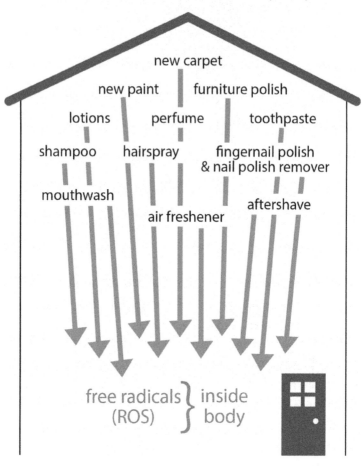

The Environmental Protection Agency (EPA) has been charged with providing guidelines and protection for the American public. They have suggested maximum levels of toxic substances in air and water. Unfortunately the studies are done on isolated substances, and no studies are done on the cumulative damage of multiple chemical exposures at low "safe" doses.

In the world of toxicity testing, the lethal dose represents the most reliable outcome measurement. Lethal dose 50 (LD50) means that 50% of the test animals died at that dose. LD100 means that 100% of the test animals died at that dose, and LD10 means 10% of test animals died at that particular dose. In this way a "safe" dose with an LD of 0 can be determined.

It is much more difficult to test and assess the dose of multiple toxic substances at "safe" doses that add up to cause an LD50 or LD10. Each "safe" level substance produces its own set of damages in the body, and the cumulative effect may be devastating.

Medication and prescription drugs all need to be metabolized and converted into substances the body can eliminate. Anti-inflammatories and diuretics are commonly used and produce ROS. Anti-cancer chemotherapeutic agents kill cancer cells through the specific use of free radicals. Unfortunately, normal cells are damaged in the process. Fortunately, some of the newer chemotherapeutic agents are targeted for specific cell types and cause less damage to normal cells. LD50 and LD100 levels on individual drugs must be submitted to the FDA prior to clearance, but research of LD levels is lacking on multiple drug use.

Foods are an important source of free radicals. Fried food is often cooked in oil that has oxidized, conferring that oxidation to the food. "Processed" foods tend to have many nutrients removed. Select nutrients are added (enriched), and chemicals placed to provide flavor and color. Some of the nutrients that are removed from the food are needed for the breakdown of that food so the body is not depleted of its reserve of these nutrients, and may or may not be added back in. Chemicals in food are just another way to form ROS.

Even the breakdown of healthy fats, carbohydrates and proteins involves the movement of electrons, oxygen or hydrogen, and the formation of free radicals. In fact, 24 electrons are transferred in the process of converting glucose into oxygen and the formation of energy (ATP). Exercise and its increased production of ATP also results in an increase of ROS production.

Sources from Inside the Body

The lungs bring oxygen into the body. Ninety-eight percent of the oxygen is used to make energy (ATP) in the mitochondria. Two percent or more escapes to make free radicals, especially oxidized oxygen missing an electron.[2]

Iron is a metal that is an essential nutrient at low levels in the body. At high levels (ferritin level above 80) it becomes a catalyst for free radical production of ^-OH.[3] Copper, which

is a transition metal like iron, also produces ⁻OH at excessive
levels in the body.[4]

Difference Between Minerals and (Toxic) Metals

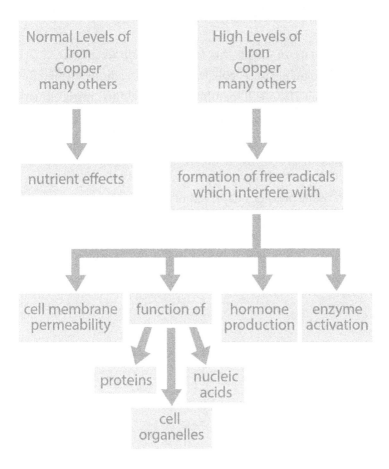

Additional transition metals include cadmium, arsenic,
mercury, chromium, beryllium, silver, nickel, antimony,

thallium. All (most?) of these metals are nutrients at low levels, but (by definition) are called "toxic metals" at high levels, when they poison the cells and interfere with normal cell and body function. This toxicity is manifest by its capability to transfer electrons, thus forming free radicals.[5]

Other transition metals that form free radicals include vanadium, manganese, cobalt, zinc. Free radicals formed by toxic metals affect cell membrane permeability, intracellular organelle functioning, structure and function of proteins and nucleic acids, formation of hormones and activation of enzymes for proper metabolism.

When tissue becomes deprived of blood with its oxygen and nutrients, it shifts to an inefficient pathway to produce energy for survival. This pathway does not require oxygen, but it does release even more free radicals.

How Lack of Oxygen Creates Massive Amounts of Free Radicals

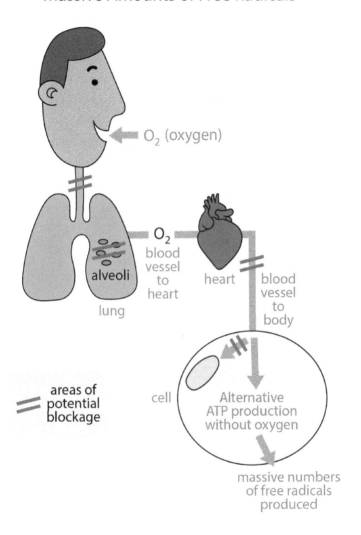

O_2 (oxygen)

O_2
blood
vessel
to
heart

alveoli

heart

lung

blood
vessel
to
body

areas of
potential
blockage

cell

Alternative
ATP production
without oxygen

massive numbers
of free radicals
produced

I have already discussed the white blood cells' use of oxygen in creating free radicals to kill microbes. There are also certain enzymes that produce ROS when they are activated to perform their tasks.

A number of chemical groups have a tendency to oxidize by themselves (auto-oxidation). These include thiols (the sulfur group on cysteine), hydroquinones, catecholamines, flavins, ferredoxins and hemoglobin. These create the oxidized oxygen (O_2^-) free radical.

Chapter Notes

1. Naidu, 101.
2. Naidu, 179.
3. Naidu, 70.
4. Naidu, 70.
5. Naidu, 69.

4

Squelching of ROS— Antioxidants

In order for signaling from ROS molecules to take place at an appropriate rate, there needs to be a way to turn off the process of ROS production and its impact in the body. When the normal signaling response is completed, it needs to be shut down. And when harmful free radicals are produced, they must be neutralized before too much damage takes place. Molecules or systems that neutralize free radicals and signaling molecules are called *antioxidants*.

Non-Enzyme Antioxidants

Glutathione is one of the most important antioxidants in the body. It is formed from 3 amino acids—cysteine, glycine, and glutamate. Cysteine has a sulfur (S-H) group that functions as the electron donor.

Glutathione is capable of quenching the lethal OH⁻ free radical, along with other oxygen-centered free radicals.

How Glutathione Squelches Free Radicals

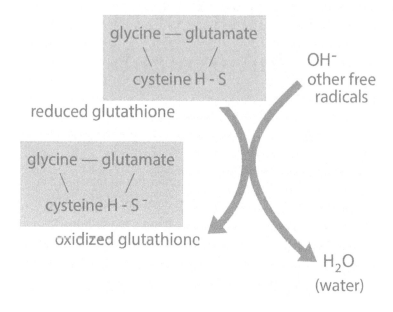

It is a good detoxification agent, especially supporting the P450 pathway in the liver, kidney, lungs, intestine and skin. There are many pathways in the body that detoxify, each one detoxifying specific toxins. P450 is one of the major pathways for medication breakdown.

Glutathione also functions as a cofactor (a substance that makes an enzyme function faster and more efficiently) in several enzyme reactions. These include *peroxidase* enzymes

REDOX CELL SIGNALING | 51

(that detoxify peroxides), *transhydoxygenase,* which improves electron transfers in NADPH and NAD$^+$, and *glutathione-S-transferase* (for conjugating estrogens and harmful xenobiotics).[1]

Uric acid is an antioxidant that resides in the blood plasma. It likewise neutralizes the toxic $^-$OH molecule. Then Vitamin C reduces the oxidized urate radical so it can reduce the next $^-$OH molecule again. Uric acid also reduces oxygen, ozone and oxidized nitric oxide.[2] Chronic excess of uric acid causes gout.

How Uric Acid Acts as an Antioxidant

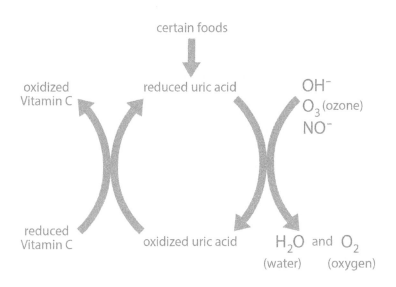

Melatonin is a small antioxidant that lives in the fat, like the

membranes of the mitochondria and nucleus. It is the best
$^-$OH free radical scavenger known, better than glutathione or
Vitamin E. It also scavengers multiple oxidized molecules,
like oxygen (O_2^-), hydrogen peroxide (H_2O_2), hypochlorous
acid, nitric oxide (NO) and ONOO$^-$.

How Melatonin Acts as an Anti-oxidant

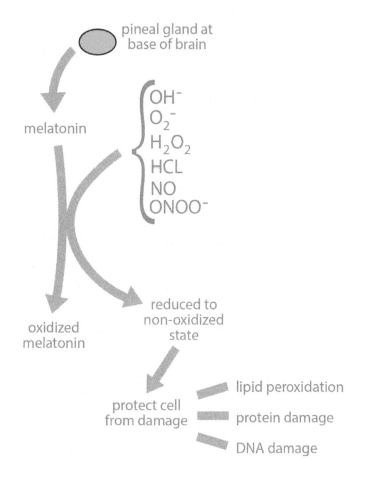

It protects cells from lipid peroxidation (cell membrane damage), protein or DNA damage. Melatonin activates other antioxidant systems including SOD, catalase, glutathione reductase, glutathione peroxidase and glucose-6-phosphate dehydrogenase.[3] It is effective in infertile women, increasing their chances of fertilization.

Enzyme Systems that are Antioxidants

Superoxide dismutase (SOD) is present in all living cells. In combination with certain metals (copper, manganese, iron, nickel), it reduces the oxidized oxygen molecule (O_2^-). The metal is now in the oxidized state. Two hydrogen molecules then attach to the oxidized metal—SOD complex which reduces the metal and releases the signaling molecule H_2O_2. This represents a wonderful system to take a highly toxic oxidized molecule and convert it into a non-toxic signaling molecule. The SOD antioxidant enzyme requires copper and zinc as cofactors in the cytoplasm and extracellular space.

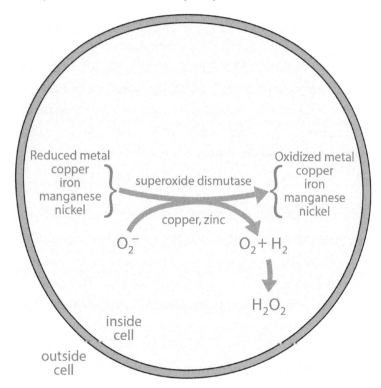

The SOD in the mitochondria requires manganese as a cofactor.[4] You might remember that cofactors are substances that are needed for enzymes to function at their best.

Catalase is another antioxidant enzyme that converts millions of molecules of H_2O_2 into H_2O (water) each second. This enzyme contains 4 iron groups (heme) that are electron donors.[5]

Catalase Reduces Hydrogen Peroxide

$$2\,H_2O_2 \xrightarrow{\text{catalase}} 2\,H_2O + O_2$$

Peroxidase enzymes convert hydrogen peroxide (H_2O_2) into water, leaving an oxidized glutathione or vitamin C after they donate an electron.

Peroxidase Reduces Hydrogen Peroxide

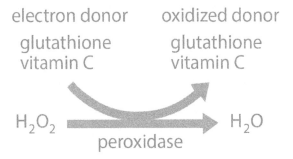

electron donor   oxidized donor
glutathione   glutathione
vitamin C   vitamin C

$H_2O_2 \xrightarrow{\text{peroxidase}} H_2O$

There are several subcategories of peroxidase enzymes. Halo-peroxidases are a subcategory of peroxidases that cause oxidation of the halide chemical groups chloride, bromide and iodide. If you look at the chemistry chart of elements, all the halides are in a row, called a "family." Thyroid peroxidase is found in the thyroid gland and is important in producing thyroid hormones, triiodothyronine (T_3) and thyroxine (T_4). The 3 in T3 and 4 in T4 refers to the number of iodine molecules on each hormone. Lactoperoxidase is secreted from the mammary gland or salivary tissue to use the halide chemicals to oxidize "bullets" for anti-microbial activity. Myeloperoxidase is found in neutrophils (WBC). It uses iron as a cofactor to oxidize and kill microbes.[6] It imparts the green color to pus.

Antioxidant Vitamins

Ascorbic acid is the most studied and utilized part of Vitamin C. It is water soluble and is an electron donor for eight enzymes. It can regenerate oxidized Vitamins E and A back into the reduced state.

How Vitamin C reduces oxidized Vitamin E and A

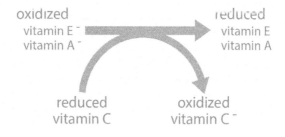

Ascorbic acid protects LDL from oxidation, which is the toxic LDL that contributes to plaque and vascular disease.

LDL Protection from Vitamin C

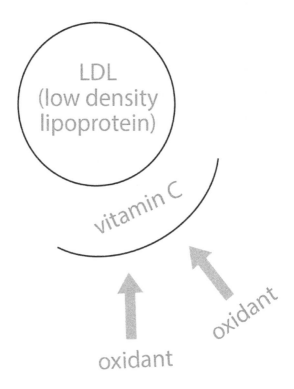

It also reduces general oxidation in the intestinal tract. It is needed for the proper "folding" of some proteins to help stabilize them. If proteins are not folded properly, they cannot function.

Ascorbic acid is needed as a cofactor for enzymes (hydroxylases, monooxygenases) that make collagen, neurotransmitters and carnitine. Collagen is the protein connective tissue that holds the body together. It is found in bones, muscles, skin, and tendons. Neurotransmitters are the communication system in the brain and intestinal tract. Carnitine is the carrier protein that transports triglycerides into the mitochondria to be broken down for energy production.

Ascorbic acid is involved in the process of converting cholesterol into bile acids for fat digestion from the gall bladder. It is also the catalyst needed in the production of *oxytocin, vasopressin, cholecystokinen* and *α-melanotropin*.[7] Oxytocin is a hormone and neurotransmitter involved with childbirth and breast feeding. It is part of maternal-child bonding, and is released with hugging, kissing and sexual relations. *Vasopressin* (anti-diuretic hormone) has to do with salt and water regulation in the kidney. *Cholecystokinin* is released from the beginning of the small intestine (duodenum) and causes gall bladder contraction for release of bile acids and digestive enzyme release from the pancreas. *Alpha-melanotropin* is a hormone that helps regulate appetite, food intake and energy production.

As you can see, Vitamin C is necessary for many more functions than just its oxidation/reduction role.

Alpha-tocopherol is one of four tocopherols in the Vitamin E family, along with four tocotrienes in the family. Alpha-tocopherol is lipid soluble and is found in the unsaturated phospholipid layer of cell membranes of each cell and organelle. In fact, free radicals react 1,000 times faster with Vitamin E than they react to phospholipids. This offers tremendous protection for the cell and organelle membranes from lipid peroxidation. When Vitamin E is oxidized, Vitamin C donates its electron to reduce it. It also plays a vital role in the glutathione peroxidase pathway.[8]

Carotenoids are composed of *carotenes* (α-carotene, β-carotene and lycopene) and *xanthophylls* (zeaxanthine and lutein). The xanthophylls are important for a functioning macula (that area of the retina that sees fine detail), and helps prevent macular degeneration.

Xanthophylls Protect Macula

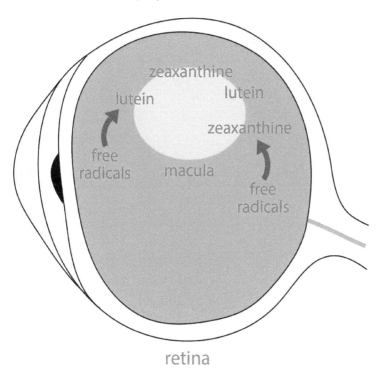

All the carotenoids function as very effective antioxidants, especially with oxidized oxygen (O_2^-), OH^- and ROO^-. Lycopene donates an electron to O_2^-. The oxidized lycopene is reduced through vibrational interactions in the tissue.

How Lycopene Reduces Free Radicals

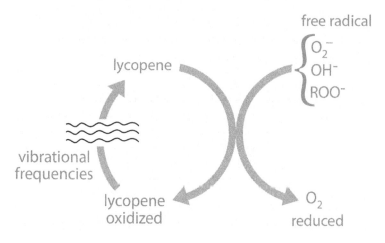

Beta-carotene is composed of two Vitamin A molecules bonded together. When the bond is broken through an enzyme process, Vitamin A is released. Vitamin A is a much less effective antioxidant compared with β-carotene.

Difference between B-carotene and Vitamin A

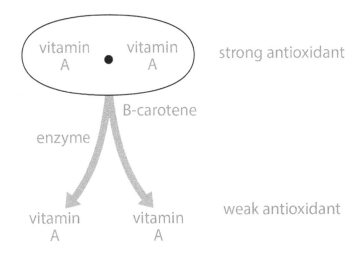

Vitamin A does protect the respiratory tract from the toxic effects of air pollution and exhaust. It is best known for its support of visual acuity, but is also helpful to resist microbes, support bone growth, immune function and fertility.[9]

Chapter Notes

1. Naidu, 144-145.
2. Naidu, 145.
3. Naidu, 146-147.
4. Naidu, 139-140.
5. Naidu, 140.
6. Naidu, 141.
7. Naidu, 147-148.

8. Naidu, 149.
9. Naidu, 150.

5

The Imbalance of Excessive ROS Oxidative Stress

Oxidative stress is the term we give to a body that has excessive ROS molecules that cannot be squelched fast enough by the antioxidant systems. The most harmful of all ROS molecules is the hydroxyl molecule, OH^-, which does the same damage in the body as ionizing radiation (like X-rays). However, when the less harmful ROS molecules overwhelm the body, damage also takes place. The 3 major attack points in the body are DNA, lipids and proteins.

How Oxidative Stress Takes Place

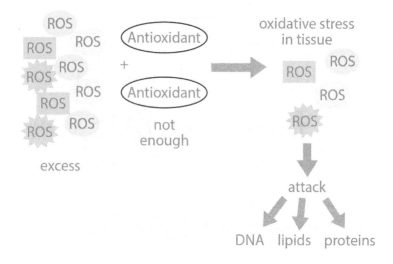

Attack on DNA

The DNA molecule is composed of two strands bound together like a twisting ladder called a *helix*. Two molecules of DNA, *guanine* and *adenine* (purines) always bind together and are across from each other in the ladder. Two other molecules, *cytosine* and *thymine* (pyrimidines), bind to each other. It is the order of the bound cells that impart the DNA code on the chromosomes.

The DNA inside each nucleus of the cell is under constant attack from oxidation. These attacks may modify the DNA base, break the DNA bond, or damage the DNA repair system. Guanine at the C-8 position is especially sensitive to ROS damage. These modifications may cause mutations to the cell, which may be part of the evolutionary process or create damaged cells that are harmful. The cell may sense the damage and stop cell reproduction so that DNA repair can take place. If the damage is too great, it will trigger a cascade to kill the cell, called *apoptosis*.[1]

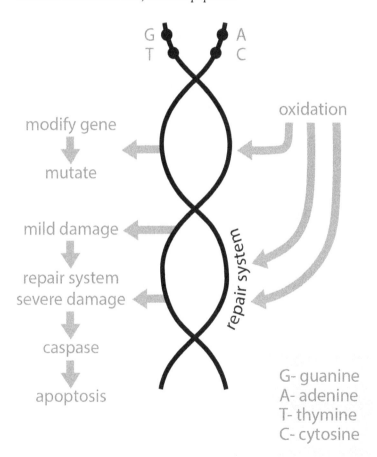

Attack on Lipids

Lipids (fats) are an important component of every cell. Every cell membrane is composed of three lipids on one end with a phosphate group (PO_4) on the other end, called a phospholipid. The lipid side loves to be with other fat molecules, while the phosphate group loves to be around water.

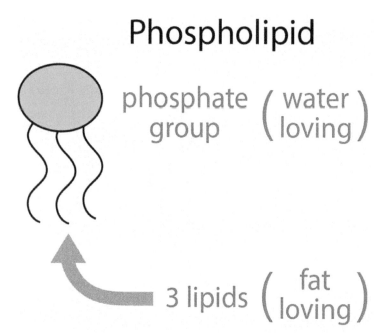

Phospholipid

phosphate group $\left(\begin{array}{c}\text{water}\\\text{loving}\end{array}\right)$

3 lipids $\left(\begin{array}{c}\text{fat}\\\text{loving}\end{array}\right)$

They form a row, with the lipid molecules all on one side and the phosphate groups on the other side. (It reminds me of a junior high dance with the girls on one side of the dance floor and the boys on the other.) When two rows are back to back with both lipid sides in the middle and the phosphate groups on the outside, the resultant formation is called a *lipid bilayer.* A continuous spherical sheet of these lipid bilayers surround the cell, called the *cell membrane.* Contained within the cell membrane are receptors (thyroid, insulin, hormone), channels (that open and close to let things in and out), cholesterol (as a strong antioxidant).

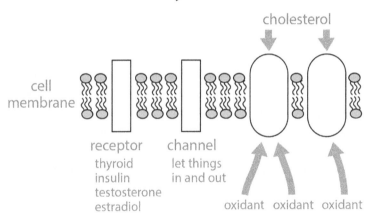

Normal Level of Oxidants are Reduced by Cholesterol

The decision of what goes on inside the cell is made at the cell membrane level (and not the nucleus).

When the oxidative stress/ROS molecules run rampant, and exceed the cholesterol antioxidant activity, the lipids in the cell membrane oxidize. We call this *lipid peroxidation.*

Oxidative Stress Overwhelms the Cholesterol Antioxidants Causing Lipid Peroxidation

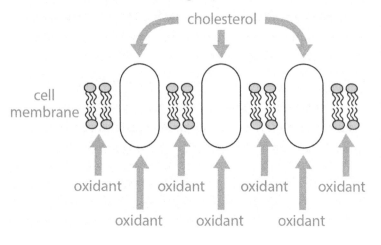

Oxidized lipids trigger a chain reaction that forms harmful aldehydes. Malondialdehyde attacks DNA and causes gene mutations. Another aldehyde, 4-OH-2-nonemal, will attack proteins. Hydrogen peroxide is also formed.[2]

As the cell membrane breaks down, the cell no longer functions. When the membrane around the organelles breaks down, the cell cannot perform that particular function. As more and more cells break down, it causes tissue breakdown, followed by organ breakdowns and dysfunction. Ultimately the body breaks down. This is called *degeneration*.

Attack on Proteins

Proteins are made up of amino acids. Enzymes are made of proteins. Proteins also make up the channel transport system in the cell membrane.

Amino Acids combine to form various Proteins

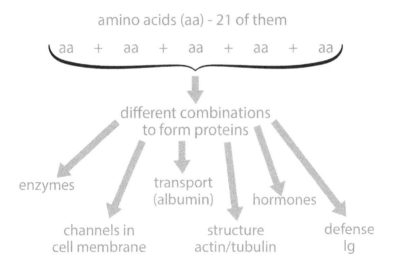

amino acids (aa) - 21 of them

aa + aa + aa + aa + aa

different combinations
to form proteins

enzymes

transport
(albumin)

hormones

channels in
cell membrane

structure
actin/tubulin

defense
Ig

Some amino acids that have sulfur-hydrogen (S-H) groups are more susceptible to oxidation—like cysteine and methionine. The transport system stops functioning when proteins oxidize. Some of the oxidative changes are reversible and others, using nitrogen as the oxidant, are irreversible. Not only can the amino acids be damaged; alterations can take place in the protein structure. The protein can degrade or fragment, all of which alters its function. When the enzymes no longer function, ATP (energy) production reduces, and altered protein in the cell membrane interferes with its ability to function.

Oxidative Stress Effect on Proteins

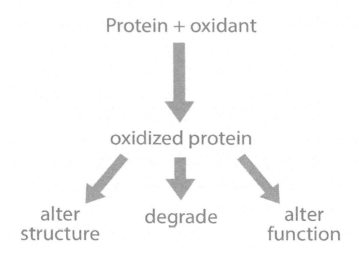

Other amino acids are sensitive to metals and cause oxidation—lysine, arginine, histidine, proline, threonine are among those amino acids catalyzed by metals.[3]

As oxidative stress accelerates and cascades forward, there is yet another way to cause oxidation. An oxidized molecule may combine with another molecule, making the new combined molecule oxidized.

Oxidant May Combine With Another Molecule Forming One Oxidized Molecule

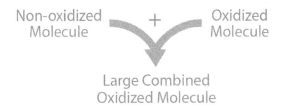

Non-oxidized Molecule + Oxidized Molecule

Large Combined Oxidized Molecule

There is no exchange of electrons, but this combination of molecules is called an adduct. These adducts can go on to oxidize proteins, or lipids, or even cause harmful carbohydrates, called *glycation*. (Glycation is the process by which a glucose molecule combines with cells or tissue and causes damage because they are sticky and inflammatory.) These big oxidant molecules further damage proteins or result in cell death.

Oxidation by Metals

Certain metals, both "toxic" and transition metals participate in the oxidation process. "Toxic" metals are only classified as toxic when they are harmful to the body. Many of these metals are critical for normal body function. These metals include copper, iron, cadmium, arsenic, mercury, chromium, antimony, beryllium, thallium, silver, and nickel. All these metals are capable of transferring electrons. Transition metals are more stable, but are still capable of creating free radicals. These metals include scandium, titanium, vanadium, chromium, manganese, iron, cobalt, nickel, copper, and zinc.

These metals all participate in ROS production with resulting affect on cell membrane permeability, organelle membrane permeability and function. They can affect the structure and function of proteins and nucleic acids (DNA). Oxidation of metals interferes with the formation of hormones, the function of enzymes and interferes with all metabolic processes.[4]

You can see that the out-of-control free radicals/ROS will cause the breakdown of every cell, tissue, organ and eventual health of the whole body. This process is called *degeneration* of the body, and accelerates the aging process. In fact, 95% of all adult disease is degenerative disease. This is caused by oxidative stress (increased production of ROS/free radicals) with age.

Ultimate Endpoint of Oxidative Stress

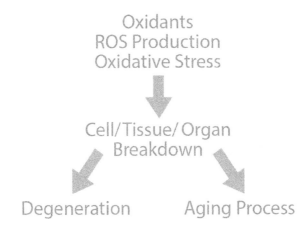

In fact, three of the major theories of aging center around REDOX reactions   The most compelling theory of aging is that oxidative stress and its ability to interfere with all the processes of the body accelerates aging.

The second theory of aging revolves around the breakdown of the mitochondria that are necessary to make the energy to fuel the needs of the cell.

The third theory of aging centers on the reduction of signaling molecules with age. Without the proper signaling, repair can't take place, cell mutations cannot be destroyed, communication between cells and within cells is diminished. Any or all of these theories are certainly a big part of normal aging.[5]

The good news is there are things we can do, eat and take

into our bodies to slow down this aging process by REDOX reactions.

Chapter Notes

1. Naidu, 108.
2. Naidu, 106.
3. Naidu, 107.
4. Naidu, 68-71.
5. Naidu, 156-160.

6

Solutions for a
Healthy REDOX Life

The simplified version of how to have a healthy REDOX
life is to:

1. Bring into the body fewer poisons, toxins and oxidized
   substances.

2. Bring into the body more nutrients and antioxidants.

3. Bring into the body more REDOX signaling molecules
   to enhance all processes in the body.

Nutrients and Antioxidants

We live in a fast-paced society and want everything now, or
yesterday. This includes shorter introductions to songs,
shorter commercials, fast-paced action in movies, fast food,
fast transportation. However, this pace may lead to an un-

healthy lifestyle, which includes accelerated aging and body breakdown.

What do we need to bring into our bodies so our cells can thrive and perform their proper functions? At the biochemical level, metabolism takes place through a series of reactions, some of which require enzymes to move the reaction forward. In order for enzymes to work efficiently, they need additional cofactors. These cofactors that assist the enzymes are vitamins and minerals that we ingest. Each enzyme needs its own specific cofactors to make it work.

Remember when we talked about the antioxidant superoxide dismutase (SOD)? Inside and outside the cell, SOD needs copper and zinc to function, and inside the mitochondria it needs manganese. If these minerals are lacking, SOD does not function well and ROS builds up inside and outside the cell.

There are thousands of these biochemical reactions throughout our body, each one requiring its own specific vitamin or mineral or molecule for the execution of its task. For example, over 300 reactions require magnesium,[1] over 140 reactions require B6[2] and over 100 reactions require B12.

Food is our source of these nutrients.[3] However, the quality of various foods differs greatly. Vegetables and legumes are the most nutrient dense with vitamins and minerals. Of course, the food is only as good as the ground it is raised in. If minerals are deficient in the soil, they will not be drawn up into the plant. Hence the importance of rotating crops in the same soil. Different crops need different nutrients. Nutrients can be added to the soil. Unfortunately, many crop producers are more focused on substances that make the plant grow or turn the proper color while ignoring the importance of micronutrients.[4]

With the transportation of food across the country, some food is harvested early so it won't spoil before getting to market. This is before all the nutrients would have been drawn into the plant. Sometimes a chemical is sprayed on the food to slow down ripening.[5] (Oops, I am getting ahead of myself, talking about toxins before their turn.)

When we talk about the nutritional value of vegetables and fruits, fresh is always best, while frozen is a close second. Old fresh may not be as good as frozen, but is generally much better than canned. Canned foods tend to have the nutrients cooked out of them, although the food industry often adds 'nutrients' at the end and calls the resulting product 'enriched.' Organic is the best, although the definition of organic is changing (as with everything that was pure and unadulterated).

Whole grains have nutrients (especially B vitamins) in the outer hull to assist the body in digesting the carbohydrate center. If the outer hull has been polished off, the body needs to draw on its reserve of B vitamins to facilitate digestion. Eventually there will be a B vitamin nutrient deficiency state if it is not corrected.[6]

There are many sources to ingest proteins. In order for

meat to be a good source, it is best that beef and poultry are free range and organic or vegetarian fed. Seafood is best from the deep sea and clean water. Legumes are another good source of proteins, including beans, peas, and lentils.

Natural cheese and plain yogurt carry the whey (cows milk) protein without the processing that milk goes through. Milk is pasteurized to kill microbes, but it denatures enzymes and nutrients in the process. Raw milk has not been processed with pasteurization, and is more healthy. However, careful cleanliness standards must be met or milk can carry harmful microbes.

Eggs are a great source of protein and fat as the antioxidant cholesterol. Free range, organic and vegetable fed chickens have healthier eggs than those of chickens raised in "concentration camps."[7] Nuts and seeds have proteins, fats and carbohydrates in them. Raw is usually best.

The topic of fats and oils could take up a whole chapter, or a whole book. We need both saturated and unsaturated fats in our body. In fact, the lipid bilayer of the cell membrane is composed of three prongs from a glycerol base. (The glycerol base is like a 'threek' with three prongs as opposed to a 'fork' which has four prongs.) Each prong has either a saturated fat or an unsaturated fat on the end.

Need for Healthy Saturated Fats and Unsaturated Fats

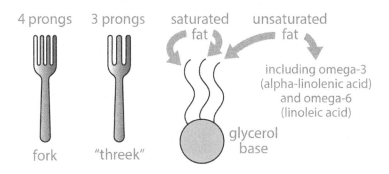

4 prongs

3 prongs

saturated fat

unsaturated fat

including omega-3
(alpha-linolenic acid)
and omega-6
(linoleic acid)

fork

"threek"

glycerol base

Saturated fats are contained in animal fats and palm oil. Unsaturated fats are typically labeled by where the 'unsaturation' occurs—omega 3 site, omega 6 site, omega 9 site, etc. Saturated fats are more stable because the unsaturated fats can oxidize at the unsaturated site. Fat oxidation is called *rancidity*. Unsaturated fats oxidize at different temperatures, so one must be careful using olive oil above 400° F. Coconut oil is more stable for cooking without oxidizing. Butter is more stable still.[8]

Temperatures at which Certain Oils Oxidize

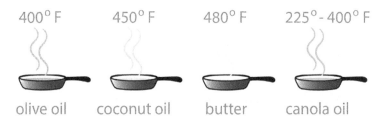

400° F

450° F

480° F

225° - 400° F

olive oil

coconut oil

butter

canola oil

When oil smokes, it is oxidizing. (Think of the oil french fries are cooked in.)

The omega-3 parent compound (α-linolenic acid) and omega-6 oils are the most important unsaturated fats in the cells membrane. Omega-3 downstream oils (EPA and DHA) are the fish oils which help with inflammation, while flax-seed is the parent compound of the omega-3 which helps form the lipid bilayer of the cell membrane. The omega-6 oils are borage oil, evening primrose oil and sesame seed oil.

It is almost impossible to get all the nutrients we need from even the best of food. We need additional nutrients because of all the toxins we are exposed to, depleted soil, and early harvesting.[9]

We all need supplements as an important aspect of insuring adequate or especially optimal vitamin and mineral status. Also, because we all have different nutrient needs, one person will need an excess of a certain nutrient, while another needs a different nutrient. This is called *biochemical individuality*.[10]

Biochemical Individuality

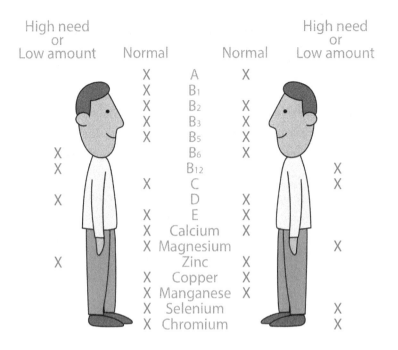

As if this were not enough, some nutrients can be made in the body, but not in the amount necessary for optimal health. Some nutrients are produced less and less with age. These are called *conditional nutrients*, as they may be enough in some circumstances, but insufficient in times of stress or greater need.[11]

Everyone should be taking certain supplements. These include:

1. A multivitamin that has the known mineral and vitamin micronutrients and macronutrients present, along with the antioxidant vitamins of C, E, carotenes and vitamin A. Although not mentioned previously, many of the minerals have antioxidant properties.

2. Vitamin D has risen to the forefront with research on its many properties-especially with immune boosting. Levels needed to boost the immune system cannot be obtained from food sources alone. Vitamin D receptors are found throughout the body, including brain and heart.

3. Fish oils and flaxseed oils (Omega-3) cannot be made in the body, so they must be ingested.

4. Omega-6 oils also must be supplemented because the body doesn't produce them.

5. I would add a good probiotic to the above recommended list of supplements everyone should be taking.

6. Phytonutrients comprise another important category of nutrients. They mostly come from fruits, but also come from vegetables, grains, and oils. They carry a high concentration of antioxidants and other health-promoting properties, and may be found as part of a multivitamin or taken separately.

Suggested Supplements for Everyone to be Healthy

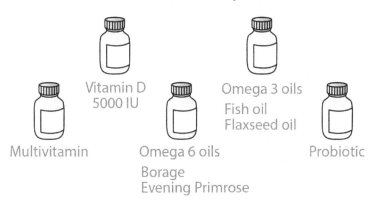

Vitamin D
5000 IU

Omega 3 oils
Fish oil
Flaxseed oil

Multivitamin

Omega 6 oils
Borage
Evening Primrose

Probiotic

Reduce the External Triggers of Oxidation

The purpose of this section is to create awareness of the many sources of harm to our body so we can make a conscious effort to reduce or eliminate as many as we can.

Let's start with a continuation of how food contributes to oxidative stress. Organic (as defined years ago) food has the nutrients we need. In order to reduce spoilage and keep things on the shelf for retail sale, many foods have been processed and placed in a can or box. The processing of food typically removes up to 80% of nutrients. The food industry replaces a few nutrients and calls it 'enriched' or 'fortified.' Processed foods tend to be high in sugar, trans fats, sodium and additives.[12]

The Difference Between Real Food and Processed Food

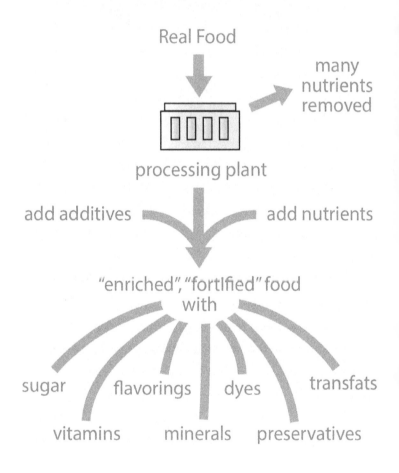

White refined sugar has had all of its nutrients and fiber stripped from it. When ingested, it is absorbed rapidly, as there is no fiber to slow down absorption. It is highly inflammatory and causes insulin resistance. Insulin resistance happens when the blood sugar remains high because insulin is no longer efficient at taking glucose into the cell. Both high insulin (the most inflammatory substance the body makes) and high sugar damage the body. In fact, high sugars start sticking to other cells, like the kidney, blood vessels, eyes, or red blood cells; a process called *glycation*. These sticky cells interfere with normal cell function.

One Danger of Ingesting Refined Sugar

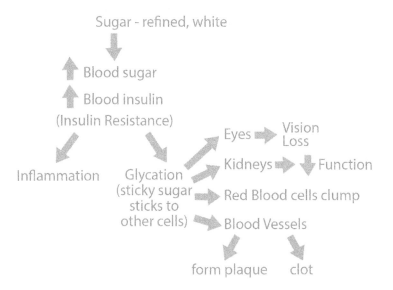

Behavioral changes take place as the sugar levels in the blood rise rapidly. I theorize (with good reason) that this is why the school system has their Halloween parties at the end of the day, so they can send the children home for their parents to deal with them. Cancer cells and yeast (candida) feed off sugar in the bloodstream.[13]

One way the body reduces blood sugar level is by converting it into *triglycerides*, which is an independent risk factor for heart disease. Sugar addiction is just as real as alcohol or cigarette addiction, and more difficult to overcome because sugar is everywhere in our society.

Because unsaturated fats in food oxidize (turn rancid) on the shelf, it has a shorter shelf life. The food industry discovered that if they hydrogenate the oil (run hydrogen through it), they could create a partially or fully hydrogenated oil that would not go rancid. This means it could stay on the shelf 'forever.' It is called a *trans fatty acid*.

What Happens with Healthy Unsaturated Oils

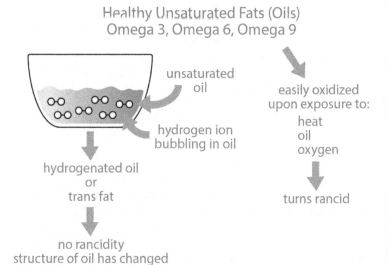

Healthy Unsaturated Fats (Oils)
Omega 3, Omega 6, Omega 9

unsaturated oil

hydrogen ion bubbling in oil

hydrogenated oil
or
trans fat

no rancidity
structure of oil has changed

easily oxidized upon exposure to:
heat
oil
oxygen

turns rancid

Unfortunately, the lipid bilayer of the cell wall cannot differ-entiate between a healthy saturated and healthy unsaturated fat and an unhealthy trans fat. It will put either one on the 'threek' of the glycerol base. The more trans fats there are in the cell membrane wall, the more stiff the wall becomes and does not function well.[14]

Additives are placed into food for a variety of reasons. The term additives is just a nice name for chemicals. There are a limited number of companies in the US that make chemicals that carry the frequencies for taste and smell. Perfumes are created in a similar manner. The right chemical can make most any food taste 'better.' MSG, or monosodium gluta-mate, has enhanced the flavor of food for centuries. Unfortunately, in susceptible individuals it interferes with the sodium and calcium transport at the cell membrane. This *excitotoxin* contributes to degeneration in the brain.[15]

Another category of 'additive' contributes to a longer shelf-life for a product. These are called *preservatives.* All of these are chemicals, and many are toxic to the body.[16]

In order to make a product appeal to the eye, chemical dyes of various colors are added. Many of these dyes cause allergies, thus making them toxic to the body:[17]

1. Soda pop has so many harmful effects. We have already talked about sugar as a sweetener and its harmful effects. Worse than sugar is the sweetener

substitute aspartame. Aspartame is a wood alcohol that the body converts into toxic formaldehyde and finally formic acid, which is the sting of the fire ant.

2. Soda pop tends to be acidic, which adds to the total body load of acid. More acid in the body encourages microbes to multiply, and is the milieu necessary for cancer cells to thrive.

3. A phosphate buffer added to soda pop reduces the harmful impact of acidity. But high phosphorus levels in the body cause heart disease, kidney disease and accelerate aging.[18]

4. When coca-cola was first introduced to the market, its name was derived from the ingredient which it contained, cocaine. When cocaine was outlawed in the drink, another addictive substance replaced it— caffeine.[19] Caffeine is not only addictive, but it also causes inflammation, is a stimulant to the brain, and is a diuretic.[20]

Harmful Effects of Soda Pop

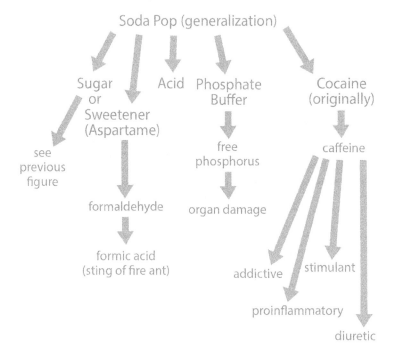

We have already talked about the kind of meat that is optimal to eat. Now let's address the problems with meat. Beef is often fed in concentration camp like conditions. In these conditions the animals are susceptible to infections, so antibiotics are given, which are found in the meat. Cows are sent to butcher as young as possible before the manifestation of neurologic breakdown from the Crutzfeld-Jacob prion. Because beef is sold by weight, growth hormones and testosterone are often added to the feed, all of which may be present in the meat we eat.[21]

Process of Beef Production

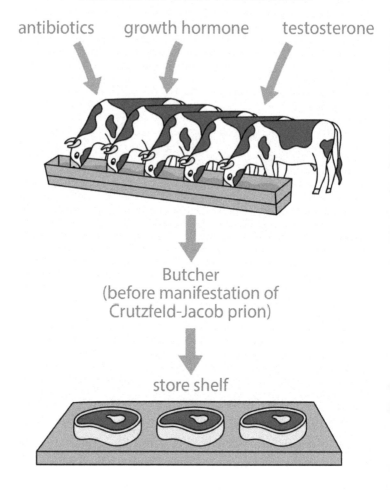

antibiotics   growth hormone   testosterone

Butcher
(before manifestation of
Crutzfeld-Jacob prion)

store shelf

Poultry is often raised in concentration camp-like conditions. The feed chickens were given used to have arsenic in it, to suppress microbe growth and encourage weight gain. Arsenic has been banned since 2013 in the poultry feed, although other countries may still use it. We should be careful in consuming imported meats.

Mercury remains an issue with ingestion of fish. We pollute the air with mercury and other toxic substances, which land in the water. Plankton takes up the toxin, which is eaten by small fish. The small fish are eaten by medium sized fish, which are eaten by big fish. This pollutes all seafood.[22]

How Seafood is Contaminated with Mercury

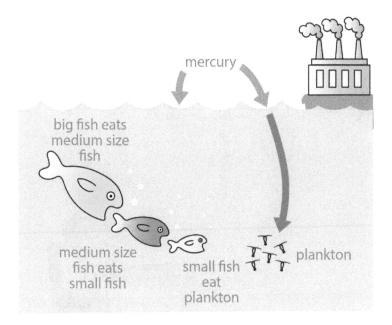

Fields of produce are sprayed with pesticides, in order to reduce the 'pests' that get into the crop. Pesticides are chemicals that have been found to interfere with the metabolic processes of the pest enough to kill them. In order to keep the weeds under control, herbicides are sprayed. These chemicals are designed to be more toxic to the weeds than they are to the crop. All these chemicals are present on the food, and may penetrate the food.

How We Ingest Toxins

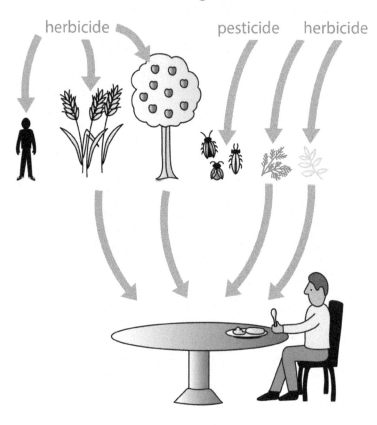

Be sure to rinse fruits and vegetables well before eating. Herbicides and pesticides drain through the soil and end up in the aquifer (our water supply). "Safe" toxin levels are permitted in tap water. There are multiple water filtration systems which help to reduce toxic load in the water.

Cookware contents can be harmful to us. Teflon emits a poisonous gas when it gets to temperatures above 680° F.[23] Aluminum pans and castiron cookware may both release their contents into the food. Aluminum and lead are both harmful to the brain.[24] Use other cookware.

More Sources of Toxins

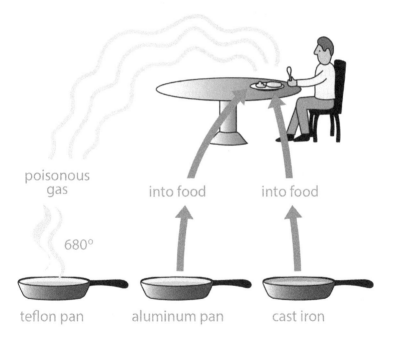

poisonous gas

680°

into food

into food

teflon pan

aluminum pan

cast iron

Most personal care products are filled with toxic ingredients. The most common include:

- Phthalates, CEP, DBP to hold color and scent; these are endocrine disruptors

- Parabens act as a preservative, suppressing bacteria and fungus; they disrupt hormones and mimic estrogen

- Sodium lauryl/laureth sulfate are used as a surfactant (reduce surface tension) and emulsifier (stabilizes the active particles in solution) and detergent (latherability); they contain 4-dioxane, a contaminant which causes cancer, nerve damage, reproductive disruption

- Polyethylene glycol (PEG), most often used for thickening, cleansing, and surfactant; may cause allergic reactions and opens pores so toxins can enter skin more readily

- Propylene glycol is used for conditioning; causes allergies, is irritating to the skin

- MEA, DEA, TEA (mono-, di-, tri-ethanolamine) is used as an emulsifier and foaming agents, adjust pH; may cause allergic reactions, dry skin

- Hydantoin and urea used for preservative; may release formaldehyde and cause allergic skin reactions

- Colors, pigments for coloring; may cause skin irritation

- Chemical sunscreens to block UVB rays; may disrupt endocrine system and release free radicals.[25]

- Personal care products include shampoos, lotions, fingernail polish and remover, toothpaste, mouth-wash, hair spray, aftershave, perfume.

There are organic products without these toxins. Don't feel overwhelmed to the point of inaction, ridding your body of toxins. Work on finding organic options one by one, thereby reducing your toxic exposure load.

Personal Care Products with Toxins

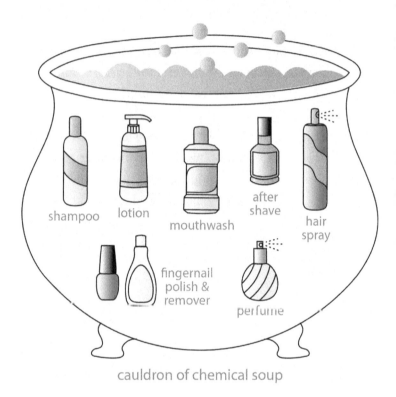

shampoo   lotion   mouthwash   after shave   hair spray

fingernail polish & remover   perfume

cauldron of chemical soup

We spend most of our time at home, where air quality is generally worse than the pollution outside (including inversion air). There is outgassing of new furniture , carpets and paint —leave the doors and windows open and use fans. Change filters on the furnaces and air conditioning units frequently.

Although dentists are not filling teeth with mercury as much as they did 20 years ago, be sure your dentist is putting in white porcelain or composite resins that don't contain mercury.

Several toxic metal chelators pull toxic metals out of the tissue so the body can remove it. Two herbs that chelate are chlorella and cilantro. Zeolite is a strong chelator. The strongest chelators are by prescription—DMSA, EDTA, DMPS.

Several organs of the body are designed to remove toxins from the body. We can support those organs in various ways.

- Kidneys—drink at least 8 cups water per day

- Liver—supplement with milk thistle, α-lipoic acid

- Gastrointestinal tract—have at least one bowel movement per day, bind toxins in gut with charcoal or clay; colonics and coffee enemas remove toxins through bile

- Skin—far-infrared saunas to cause sweating.

Detox Organs

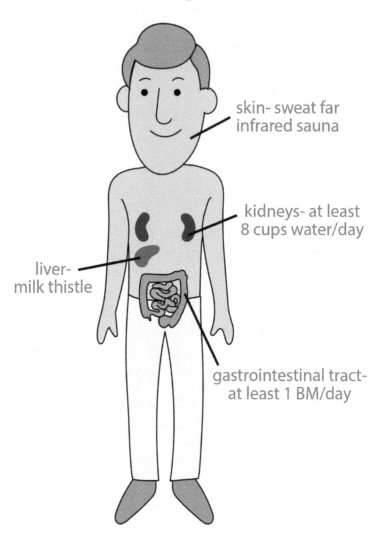

skin- sweat far infrared sauna

kidneys- at least 8 cups water/day

liver- milk thistle

gastrointestinal tract- at least 1 BM/day

A few other detox techniques include:

- Fasting for up to 3 to 5 days (just water or simple liquids)

- Energy treatments to release toxins in tissue, including acupuncture, Jin Shin Jyutsu, massage therapy, craniosacral therapy

- Glutathione is good at removing toxins from the brain and body, and functions as a good antioxidant.

Chapter Notes

1. *Magnesium in Diet* (U.S. National Library of Medicine, Medline Plus).
2. *Molecules* (U.S. National Library of Medicine, 2010 January; 15(1)), 442-259.
3. Michael Janson, MD, *The Vitamin Revolution in Health Care*
4. (Greenville, New Hampshire: Arcadia Press, 1996), 25.
5. Janson, MD, *The Vitamin Revolution*, 36-38.
6. Schneider and Norman, MD, *History of a Vitamin*, 11.
7. Cheryl Long and Tabitha Alterman, *Meet Real Free Range Eggs* , Oct/Nov 2007).
8. Anita Bancroft, (Colorado State University: Kendall Reagan Nutrition Center, April 2019).
9. Janson, MD, *The Vitamin Revolution*, 33-34.

10. Janson, MD, *The Vitamin Revolution,* 31-32.

11. Barry S. Kendler, *Supplemental Essential Nutrients in Cardiovascular Disease Therapy* (Review: J Cardiovasc Nurs., Jan-Feb 2006), 9-16.

12. Claire McArthy, MD, *Common Food Additives and Chemicals Harmful to Children* (Harvard Health Blog, July 24, 2018).

13. Jillian Kubala, MS, RD, *Eleven Reasons Why Too Much Sugar is Bad for You* (Healthline, June 3, 2018).

14. Jeremy Kaslow, MD. *Trans Fats.*

15. McArthy, MD, *Common Food Additives and Chemicals Harmful to Children.*

16. *Use of Chemicals in Food* (The Fact Factor, June 14, 2020).

17. Becky Bell, MS, RD, *Food Dyes: Harmless or Harmful?* (Healthline, Jan 7, 2017).

18. Katie Wells, *Ten Reasons to Avoid Soda (and How to Kick the Habit)* (Wellness Mama, April 16, 2018), 1.

19. Elizabeth Palermo, *Does Coca-cola contain Cocaine?* (Live Science, Dec 16, 2013).

20. *Caffeine* (WebMD).

21. Jo Robinson, *What You Need to Know About the Beef Industry* (Mother Earth News, Feb/March 2008).

22. Mary Jane Brown, PhD, PD, *Should You Avoid Fish Because of Mercury?* (Healthline, Sept 14, 2018).

23. Daisy Coyle, APD, *Is Non-stick Cookware like Teflon Safe to Use?* (Healthline, July 13, 2017).

24. *Can Cookware Be Toxic? What to Know and How to Choose Pots and Pans* (Healthline, last medically reviewed Sept 26, 2019).

25. Abigail Haynes Smith, Biological Medicine Network Manager (Marion Institute).

7

ASEA REDOX Cell Signaling Molecules and More

ASEA REDOX solution is formed through a patented electrochemical process using pure salt (NaCl) and pure water (H_2O). The elements of sodium, chloride, hydrogen and oxygen are separated and recombine during this process to form various reactive oxygen species using only those four elements. Hypochlorite (ClO⁻) is the major ROS formed.[1]*

Process of Converting Salt and Water Into ROS

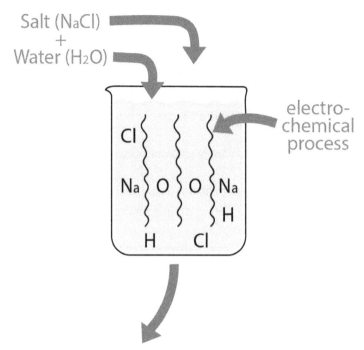

Salt (NaCl)
+
Water (H₂O)

Cl

Na O O Na
H
H Cl

electro-
chemical
process

Reactive Oxygen Species (ROS)

BioAgilytix Laboratories provides bio-analysis for third party validation of products from pharmaceutical and bio-tech companies. They validate the existence of redox signaling molecules in ASEA REDOX solution on a yearly basis.[2]*

In order to see if ASEA's signaling molecules could affect gene transcription and their positive consequences in the body, ASEA partnered with Taueret Laboratories, a leading genetic research laboratory. After an 8-week study with 60 adults, they identified five genes that increased their genetic activity from 20 to 30%. One of these genes affects 15 separate pathways. The short summary of this study shows that ASEA affected the body through gene transcription in the following ways:

- Activating the natural (innate) immune system

- Activating vascular health maintenance and elasticity

- Potential digestive health benefits through increasing enzyme production and limiting indigestion

- Hormone activation pathway activation

- Reduction in inflammation and enhanced immuno-tolerance

After the study's completion, the acceleration of those five genes returned back to baseline, further documenting the importance of regularly ingesting ASEA redox signaling molecules.[3]*

In addition to signaling all those pathways with its potential for increasing health, ASEA REDOX Cell Signaling Supplement has also been found to up-regulate antioxidants in the body. Researchers exposed human endothelial cells (the inner layer of arteries) to ASEA. Through western blot analysis, they could measure the messengers in the nucleus that activate antioxidants and found they were clearly increased.[4]*

How ASEA Redox Supplement Increases Antioxidants in Blood Vessels

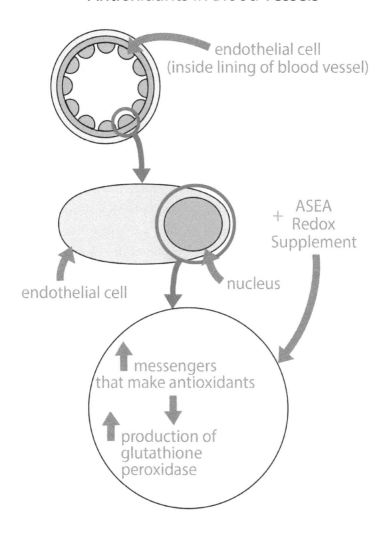

endothelial cell
(inside lining of blood vessel)

+ ASEA Redox Supplement

endothelial cell

nucleus

↑ messengers that make antioxidants

↓

↑ production of glutathione peroxidase

In normal cells, antioxidants are increased upon exposure to toxins or inflammatory substances. This is the normal reaction of cells when inflammation is present in the area--an increase in antioxidant production. This study demonstrated that the increase in antioxidants was a direct effect of ASEA REDOX Cell Signaling Supplement on the genes that increase antioxidants, and not because ASEA REDOX Cell Signaling Supplement triggered a low-grade level of inflammation.[5]*

To further assess the effect of ASEA REDOX Cell Signaling Supplement on oxidation, Dr. David C. Nieman from the North Carolina Research Campus Human Performance Laboratory completed a study with106 overweight women. They assessed the impact that ASEA REDOX Cell Signaling Supplement had on the most harmful sub-type of cholesterol, oxidized LDL. At the conclusion of the 12-week study, a reduction of oxidized LDL of 6.3% was seen, as opposed to a .9% increase in the control group. Oxidized LDL is highly inflammatory, and is a common trigger to initiate the process of plaque formation in the arteries. In order to maintain healthy arteries and heart, low oxidized LDL is critical.[6]*

As part of a safety evaluation, Dr. Nieman's group drew labs every month and found no changes in liver or kidney function. The RBC (red blood cell) counts, hemoglobin and hematocrit showed no changes during the study. There were no adverse affects reported during the 12-week study.

Their conclusion is that ASEA REDOX Cell Signaling Supplement is safe for human consumption.[7]*

Pacific Northwest National Laboratory was also commissioned to study any toxicity to eukaryotic cells upon contact with ASEA REDOX Cell Signaling Supplement. A 5% and 20% ASEA REDOX Cell Signaling Supplement solution were exposed to the cells, along with a saline-phosphate buffered solution, and a known toxin. Measurement of inflammatory cells entering the nucleus were present, as expected with the toxin, while no inflammatory response was seen with ASEA REDOX Cell Signaling Supplement or placebo. Their conclusions were that orally administered ASEA REDOX Cell Signaling Supplement does not cause inflammation.[8]*

Once the oral route of administration had been tested for efficacy and safety, and administered in millions of doses, the company looked at another delivery system. They looked at stabilizing these molecules in a gel, thereby receiving full strength REDOX molecules on the skin, rather than the dilution of molecules that come through the bloodstream. The name of this product is RENU 28.

ASEA contracted with Dermatest Research Institute in Germany which assesses the safety and efficacy of cosmetic products for the cosmetic and pharmaceutical industries. Their 5-star rating given to ASEA for their Renu-28 product is the highest level of standard for proven skin tolerance, effectiveness, and application safety.[9]*

Another study was done with RENU 28 to assess certain aspects of skin aging. Twenty adult women over the age of 45 were administered the gel product twice a day for 4 weeks. The PRIMOS 3D scanner was used for measurements of skin roughness. Cutometry assessment measured skin elasticity, and high-resolution photographs provided digital images for facial appearance comparison. In the 4-week study, skin texture improved 22%, skin smoothness improved 23% and skin elasticity improved 20%.[10]*

Dermatest did another study assessing RENU 28 on cellulite (adipose or fat lobules under the skin). Thirty women placed the product on their thighs twice a day with a 30 to 60 second massage of the cream. After the 12 week study, the following results were seen: Length of fat lobules decreased by 12% by 6 weeks and 16% by 12 weeks. The breadth of the fat lobules decreased by 11% by 6 weeks and 15% by 12 weeks.[11]*

ASEA commissioned Stephens and Associates to study RENU 28 on cell turnover in the skin. The rate at which cells replace themselves in tissue is the essence of anti-aging. Participants applied RENU 28 to one forearm twice in the morning and twice at night for 2 weeks. Then a fluorescent dye was applied to both forearms. RENU 28 was continued as before. The dye faded in the RENU 28 arm to zero in 13.2 days. The control arm took 15.3 days to zero. This represents a 16% faster surface skin cell turnover under the influence of redox signaling molecules.[12]*

ASEA then made a cream product with a more concentrated form of REDOX signaling molecules called Renu Advanced Intensive REDOX Serum. This was tested in 10 adult women 45 years of age and older. A 3D optical scanner with a structured light projection method (PRIMOS) was used to measure the skin surface images.

Measurements were taken before application of the serum and 30 minutes after, over a period of 4 weeks. Wrinkle depth under the eye as measured by the optical scanner decreased an average of 18%. No untoward reactions or irritation took place during the study.[13]*

ASEA has broadened its skin care line to include RENU 28, RENU Advanced Ultra Replenishing Moisturizer and RENU Advanced Gentle Refining Cleanser. Stephens and Associates evaluated 40 participants in an 8-week trial to evaluate the efficacy of ASEA's total skin care system on skin aging. Researchers used the Stephens Wrinkle Imaging using Raking Light (SWIRL) for their assessment of facial imagery. The participants applied the skin care system twice each day. Imagery was done prior to the study and at 4 and 8 weeks.

The results analyzed multiple areas of the face, including crow's feet, under eye, forehead and upper lip areas. The SWIRL analysis demonstrated fine lines decreased 20%, visible photo damage decreased 10% and skin smoothness improved 19%. Survey results from the participants showed the appearance of the following:

- 100% reported a visible decrease in numerous deep fine lines

- 100% reported measurable smoother skin

- 95% reported noticeably firmer skin

- 90% indicated a decrease in visible photo-damaged skin

- 90% reported more radiant skin

- 85% noted a visible decrease in number and depth of wrinkles.[14]*

Dermatest performed a hydration study with the moisturizer used in ASEA's skin care system. Nineteen males and females applied RENU Advanced Ultra Replenishing Moisturizer once per day to the face and neck. Skin moisture measurements were taken by a Corneometer at the beginning and at the conclusion of the study. No other skin care product was used on the face during this study. Corneometer analysis at the end of 4 weeks showed a 43% increase in skin moisture.[15]*

Dermatest also performed a skin sebum balance test using the RENU Advanced Gentle Refining Cleanser. Twenty adult male and female participants cleansed their face with the product for four weeks. Sebum, which is skin fat, was measured on three spots on each participant's face before the study and at four weeks. Sebumetry was interpreted by a dermatology specialist with expertise in analysis of sebum. They found a 17% decrease of sebum over four weeks.[16]*

In the world of research, the gold standard is a double-blind placebo-controlled study. A placebo arm is present in each of the above studies, but they are not double blinded. However, the research clearly establishes the safety and lack of toxicity with any of the products. Research was done on cells and animals and humans with positive results.

Because ASEA is regarded as a supplement company, it falls under the same limitations as all supplements. The FTC and the FDA insist ASEA make it clear that none of these supplements have been evaluated by the FDA, and any supplement is not intended to diagnose, treat, cure or prevent any disease.

Analysis on ASEA REDOX Cell Signaling Supplement demonstrates these signaling molecules are present in the solution. Research shows these molecules are being absorbed and having an effect on cells inside the body. ASEA is committed to research within the confines set up for the supplement community so we will have access to these revolutionary molecules for a long time to come.

These statements have not been evaluated by the Food and Drug Administration. This product is not intended to diagnose, treat, cure or prevent any disease.

Chapter Notes

1. Conversations with Scott Aldred, Vice President over Operations, ASEA, LLC. President of ASEA.

2. *Scientific Validation of ASEA Redox Supplement* (BioAgilytix Redox Certification, 2016).

3. Kenneth Ward, MD, *Initial Gene Study Showed ASEA REDOX Affected Important Signaling Pathway Genes* (ASEA, LLC. 2016).

4. *Antioxidant Up-regulation* (Scientific Validation of ASEA Redox Supplement, 2016).

5. *ASEA Redox Supplement in-vitro product safety study* (Scientific Validation, 2016).

6. *Influence of ASEA Redox Supplement Ingestion on Oxidative Stress* (Scientific Validation, 2016).

7. Nieman DC, *ASEA Metabolomics Results* (North Carolina Research Campus and Appalachian State University: David H. Murdock Research Institute).

8. *ASEA Redox Supplement in vitro product safety study* (Scientific Validation, 2016).

9. *Scientific Validation of ASEA RENU Advanced Skin Care* (Dermatest Five-Star Accreditation, 2016, ASEA, LLC.).

10. *Anti-Aging Effects of RENU 28 Revitalizing Redox Gel on Female Subjects Over age 45* (Scientific Validation of ASEA RENU Advanced Skin Care, 2016, ASEA, LLC.).

11. *Study-Effect of RENU 28 Revitalizing Redox Gel on Cellulite and Adipose Lobules* (Scientific Validation of ASEA RENU Advanced Skin Care, 2016, ASEA, LLC.).

12. *RENU 28 Revitalizing Redox Gel on Skin Turnover Renewal and Cell Turnover* (Scientific Validation of ASEA RENU Advanced Skin Care, 2016, ASEA, LLC.).

13. *Effect of RENU Advanced Intensive Redox Serum on Product Safety and Wrinkle Depth in Women 45 and Older* (Scientific Validation of ASEA RENU Advanced Skin Care, 2016, ASEA, LLC.).

14. *Effect of RENU Advanced Anti-Aging Face Care System on Human Skin* (Scientific Validation of ASEA RENU Advanced Skin Care, 2016, ASEA, LLC.).

15. *Effect of RENU Advanced Ultra Replenishing Moisturizer on Product Safety and Skin Hydration in Adult Men and Women* (Scientific Validation of ASEA RENU Advanced Skin Care, 2016, ASEA, LLC.).

16. *Effect of RENU Advanced Gentle Refining Cleanser on Product Safety and Skin Sebum Balance in Adult Men and Women* (Scientific Validation of ASEA RENU Advanced Skin Care, 2016, ASEA, LLC.).

8

ASEA Supplement Line and REDOX

ASEA has also developed supplements that are complementary with REDOX signaling molecules. Let's talk a little about supplements generally.

Supplements are ultimately under the oversight of the FDA (US Food and Drug Administration). The FDA has determined that there are no supplements that can "prevent, treat, cure" any disease or dysfunction in the body. In other words, a supplement cannot be marketed or taken by someone who is unhealthy or sick to become healthy or whole. It can only be taken by a healthy person to make them more healthy. Under FDA policy, only a drug may diagnose, prevent, treat or cure any disease.

Supplements must be ingested by mouth, and must have a disclaimer: "This statement has not been evaluated by the Food and drug Administration. This product is not

intended to diagnose, treat, cure, or prevent any disease."
Labels on supplements must be truthful and not misleading.

So, if you are a representative of any company that sells
supplements, you are limited to the above guidelines, especially in public gatherings and the internet. You may not
mention any disease state in a presentation that also men-
tions ASEA.

Supplements are commonly used in medical practitioners'
offices throughout the world to improve everyone's health.

An interesting caveat regarding disease treatment is that
most drugs that are on the market do not treat the disease
itself, but only treat the symptoms of the disease. Drugs also
control the body, rather than work with the physiology of
the body. Now let's talk about some supplement ingredients
that have a lot to do with REDOX. The rest of this chapter
is simplified from REDOX Life, previously referenced.

Vitamins

Three **vitamins** have a lot to do with REDOX. These 3
vitamins function as anti-oxidants—Vitamin A, Vitamin C,
Vitamin E.

Vitamin A is especially effective in reducing oxidants in
cigarette smoke. It also reduces oxidation in the eye,
specifically the macula. The macula is that area in the eye
that is responsible for sharp vision up close. Vitamin A

reduces the oxidative damage in the skin and provides immune system support.[1]*

Vitamin C reduces oxidants in the blood, as do all anti-oxidants. It also strengthens endothelial function, which is that thin layer on the inside of the blood vessel that is responsible for signaling and protecting the blood vessel. In addition it provides bone support and up-regulates the cell signaling of genes. [2]*

Vitamin E has a bunch of subtypes. Four are tocopherols and four are tocotrienes. They all function as Vitamin E, although the two groups have some unique properties. As a group they prevent the oxidation of the lipid membranes (fat membranes) in the body, and reduce the breakdown of unsaturated fatty acids in the body into their oxidized state. Vitamin E reduces the oxidation in wounds, and assists in the repair process. It also has the potential to prevent or reduce unsightly veins on the legs. It supports the cardio-vascular system and red blood cells, and prevents the plate-lets from clumping together.[3]*

Minerals

Several minerals have a lot to do with REDOX.

Iron is one of the minerals the body needs. At normal levels iron participates in energy production. It is necessary for oxygen binding in the red blood cells. At high levels iron is a catalyst for oxidation, which damages lipids (fats), proteins and nucleic acids (RNA and DNA). Unless we bleed (or donate blood), we cannot get rid of iron in the body. [4]*

Copper is a cofactor with zinc in *superoxide dismutase* (SOD). SOD is one of the 3 most important anti-oxidant systems in the body. In the mitochondria, copper is also needed in the last step of the electron transport chain. The electron transport chain is a multi-step process whereby most of the energy (ATP) of the body is made. This last step utilizes the enzyme cytochrome oxidase, which has two iron centers and two copper centers to permit it to function. High levels of copper are damaging to the cells. Deficiency of copper affects the nerves, muscles and blood in a negative way.[5]*

Zinc is involved in more than 300 enzymatic reactions. It works with copper in the anti-oxidant SOD (superoxide dismutase). Zinc does not oxidize or reduce, but it is involved in cell signaling.[6]*

Manganese has several oxidized states, and is a cofactor in SOD. It is also one of many minerals involved in bone metabolism, and is involved in growth. [7]*

Selenium functions as an anti-oxidant. Selenocysteine (which is selenium bound to cysteine, an amino acid) is present in five different glutathione peroxidase systems. Glutathione is touted as the most important anti-oxidant system in the body. Selenium also supports the immune system and the cardiovascular system. It is an important part of the conversion of thyroid hormone T4 into its activated state, T3.[8]*

Amino Acids

Many **amino acids** are involved in REDOX reactions. All of the amino acids can be oxidized, which modifies their proteins. The sulfur-containing amino acids are the most susceptible to oxidation. These include *cysteine* and *methionine.* Other amino acids that are highly susceptible to oxidation include *Arginine, Lysine, Proline, Histidine, Tryptophan,* and *Tyrosine.*[9]*

NAC (N-acetyl-cysteine) is an anti-oxidant and donates *cysteine,* an amino acid, to form *glutathione.* Glutathione is the major antioxidant in the body and is composed of three amino acids-cysteine, glutamate and glycine.[10]*

Methionine is an amino acid that functions as an anti-oxidant, which means it is sensitive to oxidation. It is needed to convert homocysteine into cysteine for glutathione synthesis. It assists in the absorption of zinc and selenium.[11]*

Glutamate/Glutamine is a component of glutathione, which is the major anti-oxidant system in the body. In the brain glutamine is an excitatory neurotransmitter. It is also important in the intestinal tract to maintain barrier wall function.[12]*

These statements have not been evaluated by the Food and Drug Administration. This product is not intended to diagnose, treat, cure or prevent any disease.

Chapter Notes

1. Naidu, 418-421.
2. Naidu, 422-425.
3. Naidu, 426-430.
4. Naidu, 396-398.
5. Naidu, 399-402.
6. Naidu, 403-406.
7. Naidu, 407-409.
8. Naidu, 410-414.
9. Naidu, 431-433.
10. Naidu, 434-438.
11. Naidu, 439-441.
12. Naidu, 442-445.

Frequently Asked
Questions

What is ASEA REDOX Cell Signaling Supplement?

ASEA REDOX Cell Signaling Supplement is composed of trillions of redox signaling molecules in a saline (salt) solution. These molecules are bio-identical to what the body makes.

What are REDOX signaling molecules?

There are many types of signaling molecules in the body. Some have an oxygen base and are called reactive oxygen species (ROS). They participate in the exchange of oxygen, electrons or hydrogen in a biochemical process called REDOX. There are other signaling molecules in the body whose bases are different—nitrogen and sulfur being two of them.

How do REDOX signaling molecules work?

Millions of biochemical reactions take place every second in the body. They include turning genes on and off, opening pathways for molecules to flow into and out of cells, triggering release of transmitters and hormones, receptor activation and so much more. Many of these processes are mediated through REDOX signaling molecules. It is the signal that causes things to happen, so our cells can function at their optimal level.

Is ASEA REDOX Cell Signaling Supplement approved by the FDA?

ASEA is categorized as a dietary supplement by the FDA (Food and Drug Administration). The company, ASEA, follows all current regulations and guidelines issued by the FDA. This supplement also complies with the Federal Food, Drug and Cosmetic Act. Going above and beyond that, the safety of the product is carefully researched by third party studies.

Have REDOX signaling molecules been researched?

There are many tens of thousands of articles in research journals on redox signaling, including research in various disease states. Reputable medical journals exist that are fully dedicated to this topic. ASEA has also done double-blind placebo-controlled studies performed by prestigious research facilities.

I felt worse when I started drinking ASEA REDOX Cell Signaling Supplement. How could that happen?

Most of us have absorbed or deposited toxins in our tissue. As the body starts to become more healthy, these toxins may be released from the tissue into the blood stream. We have many natural systems in our body to get rid of toxins, called our detoxification pathways. These include our kidneys (drink plenty of water), gastrointestinal tract (have daily bowel movements), skin (through sweating) and liver. If our detoxification pathways can't rid the body of these toxins fast enough, their redistribution makes us feel sick, like the flu.

Why do REDOX signaling molecules help my friend but not me, even though we have the same problem?

Even though you and your friend may have the same problem, the causes of the symptoms may be very different. Your 'cause' may take longer before you see results, or your cells may be more severely affected by the issue. You may also have other issues that require different signaling molecules to resolve your issues.

Why does my friend experience a benefit, but it does nothing for me?

In my clinical experience, it takes about a 30% response in a person before they can tell a difference. A baseline scoring system of symptoms can be very helpful in determining improvement. We tend to remember the issues that are persisting but forget about the resolved issues.

Even though REDOX signaling molecules benefit everyone who takes them, your body may also need additional molecules.

Isn't ASEA REDOX Cell Signaling Supplement just salt and water? Can I make my own solution by adding salt to water?

The production of REDOX signaling molecules (ASEA) is a patented electrochemical process that separates the sodium from chloride (salt) and hydrogen from oxygen (water). This permits the formation of new molecules, most of which are signaling molecules. This is like making a cake from scratch. The flour, sugar, eggs, oil, water and baking soda are mixed together. Through a baking process which causes chemical reactions to take place, a cake comes out of the oven which no longer resembles the original ingredients.

Why does ASEA REDOX Cell Signaling Supplement have a unique taste?

ASEA REDOX Cell Signaling Supplement is made up of salt (sodium chloride) and water (H_2O). Salt has a chloride molecule, which is different from chlorine, even though it tastes similar. Chlorine is toxic to the body, while the chloride in ASEA REDOX Cell Signaling Supplement has passed all safety and toxicity studies and is totally safe.

How much salt is in four ounces of ASEA REDOX Cell Signaling Supplement?

There are 123 mg of sodium in four ounces of ASEA. This would be the salt equivalent of eating 2 ½ large carrots. The average person ingests 2000 to 5000 mg of sodium per day, while people on a restricted salt diet typically ingest 1500 mg per day.

Glossary of Terms

Antioxidant systems—large molecules that catalyze the conversion of oxidants into reductants. The three major systems include glutathione, catalase, superoxide dismutase (SOD).

Amino acids—the building blocks of proteins. Each one has a carboxyl group (-COOH) on one end and an amine (-NH3) group on the other end. There are a total of 20 amino acids.

Electron—a negatively charged particle found outside the nucleus of matter.

Electron transport chain—series of proteins that transfer electrons to create energy (ATP). It is the major energy-producing site in the body.

Glycation—the bonding of a sugar molecule to a protein or lipid.

Homeostasis—the ability of the body or cell to maintain a condition of equilibrium or stability even when dealing with external changes.

Innate immune system—the cells that provide immediate protection from any insult to the body, including microbes. The other part of the immune system is the adaptive immune system, which includes anti-bodies that take days to form and are specific to one microbe.

Mitochondria—an organelle found in all cells that is the major pro-ducer of energy (ATP).

Oxidant—also called a free radical or reactive oxygen species. These are molecules in search of an electron. It acts as a signaling molecule and functions in killing rogue cells and unwanted microbes.

Oxidizing—the transfer of an electron from a reductant to make it an oxidant.

Oxidative stress—excessive oxidants inadequately neutralized by anti-oxidants (reductants) that cause the body to breakdown and accelerates degeneration and aging.

Phagocytes—a cell in the body which engulfs and absorbs bacteria and other cells.

Physiology—deals with the normal functions of the body.

Reactive Oxygen Species (ROS)—A type of unstable molecule that contains oxygen and that easily reacts with other molecules in tissue. They are also call free radicals.

REDOX—short for a REDuction-OXidation reaction involving transfer of electrons between molecules.

Reducing—the transfer of an electron to an oxidant to make it a stable reductant.

Reductant—a molecule that acts as an electron donor in REDOX reactions. It functions as an anti-oxidant.

CPSIA information can be obtained
at www.ICGtesting.com
Printed in the USA
BVHW010454030422
633218BV00029B/279

9 781087 981413